Acknowledgements

I would like to thank all the women in this book who have inspired me and given me their words of wisdom and depth of knowledge.

To my mentor and friend Annie Sprinkle, whose generosity of spirit and guidance has made this project possible.

To Kimberly O'Sullivan, for her invaluable help – I would not have been able to compile this book without you.

To Esmé Holmes, for her love and support.

To Ruth Ostrow, who is a wonderful friend and an inspiration.

To my brother Murray Baker, for his sense of humour and regular computer support.

To my agent David Holland, who has always steered me in the right direction.

And to Sophie Cunningham and her team at Allen & Unwin, for being there.

JO-ANNE BAKER

Contents

Introduction

Women have always been at the forefront of sexual revolution. From the feminists of the nineteenth century who fought Victorian moral hypocrisy to the present day, women have always understood the link between personal freedom and freedom of sexual expression. Often these women are forgotten, yet the names of their male counterparts – Baron von Richard Krafft-Ebing, Freud and Reich – have been immortalised in the language of sexuality. Few people would remember Victoria Woodhull or Sylvia Pankhurst who spoke out for women's sexual rights and against the social stigmatisation of sex workers and women who wished to celebrate their female eroticism.

By the 1960s women throughout the Western world had been affected by the enormous social changes of the decade. Central to those changes was an emphasis on the right to individual expression and many social freedoms, including the right to sexual freedom. With the advent of improved and more effective contraception, particularly the Pill, sex and pregnancy could be separated from each other for the first time in history.

This allowed women to take more sexual risks, to start thinking about their own sexual fulfilment, and to question traditional female roles and the nature of their relationships. However, as women started expressing their need for personal and sexual freedom they often ran into societal obstacles. Women found that, more often than not, the 1960s and 1970s ideal of an individual's right to love and live as one chose did not apply to them, and that strong social stigmas were still attached to women who were sexually free and unashamed of their desire.

The women's movement of the 1970s was a natural extension of this period as women reappraised all aspects of their lives and how they had been taught by society what a woman should be. While there was much debate and discussion about female liberation, the area of sexuality remained problematic. Over the next two decades sexual rights, responsibilities, lifestyles and choices were hotly debated. At the same time there was a group of women who identified with the earth mother archetype, the ancient goddesses and embraced a New Age philosophy of how a woman should live.

The last decade of the twentieth century has seen another sexual revolution, one based on sex positivism, the concept that sex is a healing and positive part of life. Sex positivism became an important way to counteract the hysteria around HIV/AIDS, and fight a sex-negative type of feminism that viewed sexuality as the core of women's oppression.

Sexually women have come into their own, and are talking openly about eroticism. By taking charge of their sexuality in a way that is empowering and powerful, they have changed forever how female sexuality is viewed. This newly embraced sexuality is not based on a male model, or even a traditional female one, but on a new vision. Gender roles have been explored, expanded and even discarded as women looked critically at the nature of masculinity and femininity and unravelled what was biology and what was social construction.

This new female sexuality is manifest in the many courses available on erotic massage, sadomasochism (SM), how to play with sex toys, how to make your own erotic video, striptease, breath and energy orgasm and spiritual sex. Female entrepreneurs have found a market for porn produced for women and couples, erotic products and new sex toys made to add to female sexual pleasure.

Female performance artists have publicly explored women's sexuality, putting women's intimate erotic experiences on stage in shows that are often confronting, even shocking. For other artists the new performance arena is female to male cross-dressing, with the words 'drag king' now entering the language for the first time.

For me trying to find answers to my many questions on sexuality was like searching for the Holy Grail. In that journey I met many of the women who are now profiled in this book, women who came to be (sometimes unintentionally) at the forefront of this new sexual revolution. The women in this book reflect the diversity of sexuality that is in each one of us. I respect the honesty and passion they have in their lives and the way they have used their sexuality to make a difference.

The women in this book have endured periods where they were not respected or honoured for their sexual journey. In part this book is to redress this and publicly pay tribute to the contribution they have made to creating a sex-positive world. All of the women in this book have been courageous in their fight for women's sexual rights and have often faced censure, personal attack and even threats of violence – just as their counterparts last century did.

Many of the sexual rights women take for granted were fought for by the women profiled in this book, female sexual pioneers who, for the first time, reveal their personal sexual tips and exercises. You are hearing it from the experts!

This book consists of a range of contributions: most are original interviews, some are sneak previews of yet-to-be published manuscripts, while others are sexual classics which deserve to be more widely read. The diversity of the material is deliberate as I believe that everybody's sexual journey is eclectic and individual and the contributors certainly reflect this. Some of these women's erotic journeys have been so powerful that I have included them for this reason alone.

Many of these women have influenced me directly such as my friend and mentor, Annie Sprinkle, and Jwala who, twenty years ago, introduced me to Tantra. I have always admired the work of Veronica Vera, Linda Montano, Dolores French and Joan Nestle. For years I have used Kutira's music in my workshops. Carol Queen sold me my first vibrator and dildo at Joani Blank's shop Good Vibrations, which was the inspiration for my business The Pleasure Spot.

In my shop and catalogue I have sold Candida Royalle's wonderful videos, and others starring Nina Hartley as well as Tuppy Owen's *Safer Planet Sex Handbook*. I visited Ky at Sh!, the first women's sex shop in the UK. Cora Emen runs workshops similar to mine in Amsterdam and I met Minori Kitahara when she visited Australia. Elizabeth Burton and I have had a long-time connection through her innovative strip classes for women she has taught from my business.

The women involved in SM have long fascinated me and I learned much about sexual power and trust from Cléo Dubois, Kat Sunlove and Amanda Dwyer. Performance artists Shelly Mars and Dianne Tornado have long explored gender in their work, while activist norrie mAy-welby has not only done that, but lived it.

Rosie King has been a constant support, as have my friends and peers, Ruth Ostrow and Kimberly O'Sullivan. Much of the knowledge in the public arena about female sexuality was written about by those pioneering women at *On Our Backs* magazine – Deborah

Sundahl, Nan Kinney and Susie Bright.

These women are profiled here. They also pass on their personal sexual techniques, tips and exercises which have transformed their lives, my life and those of thousands of others. These are the Pandora's box of erotic pleasure. Sit back and enjoy the ride.

1

Women Sex Performance Artists

Sex performances are as old as time. Depictions of women performing for men, or for each other, can be seen in ancient images of belly dancers in the Middle East, Indian temple performers and throughout Europe. In the nineteenth century burlesque arrived and the first striptease artists followed. In the 1870s the Folies Bergeres thrilled and scandalised Paris and in the 1920s the Ziegfeld Follies hit New York and inspired the 'flappers' craze. When the sensational Josephine Baker hit Europe, the audiences began changing from all male to couples, who saw this new entertainment as not just risqué but artistic. Erotic dancing and performance went from sleazy to bohemian and artists gained some degree of legitimacy along with their notoriety. This reflected a freeing up of women's sexuality in a society that was less rigid and more liberal. This was seen on the street where, for the first time, women's hemlines rose, they wore pants, cut their hair and smoked in public.

Two world wars saw these liberal attitudes evaporate to be followed by the post-war conservatism of the 1950s. However, in a small step toward the development of sex performance art the first peep show opened in 1950. By the 1960s society was rapidly changing as the first baby-boomers hit adolescence. In the West high employment and favourable economic conditions meant an environment where free thinking and expression of ideas was possible.

After a relaxation in the censorship laws in the 1960s, rock musicals such as *Hair* and *Oh Calcutta!* containing a high degree of nudity were performed at legitimate theatre venues. In Hollywood credible actresses were allowed to do sexual performances on film – Brigitte Bardot stripped for the camera in *And God Created Woman* in 1956, Nadia Garys stripped in *La Dolce Vita* in 1959 and Jane Fonda did a fantasy striptease in *Barbarella* in 1968.

ANNIE SPRINKLE

Something Less is More

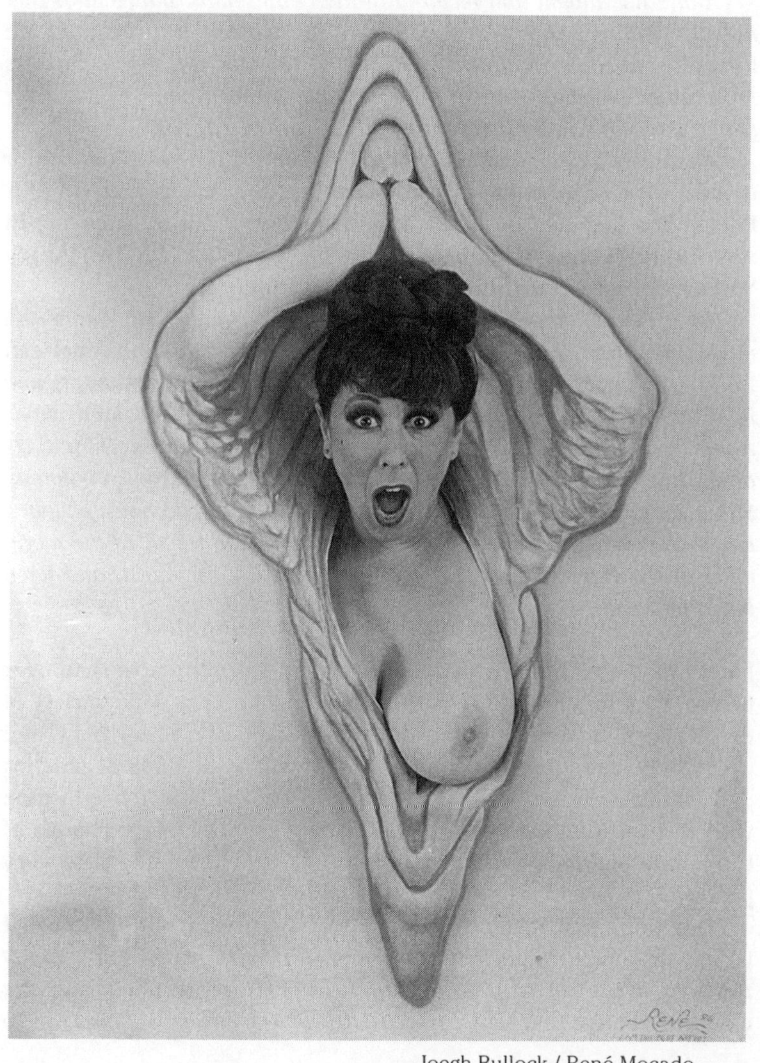

Joegh Bullock / René Mocado

Annie Sprinkle spent twenty years as a porn star, stripper and prostitute. With the advent of the AIDS crisis, she became interested in healing modalities and spirituality. She evolved into a high priestess of sacred sex magic rituals, a Tantrica, an internationally acclaimed avant-garde artist, facilitator of sex workshops, safe-sex innovator, and feminist pleasure activist. She lives on a houseboat in Sausalito, California.

Annie has taught and lectured at many museums, universities and holistic healing centres. She is one of the women who inspired the term 'sex-positive feminist' and is a founder of Pornographers Promoting Safer Sex, organised to educate pornographers to use safer sex in their film so they in turn could educate the public.

Annie has written and had published over 300 articles about sex for a variety of magazines, including Penthouse, Forum *and* On Our Backs. *She has also contributed to a number of books, including* Bi Any Other Name, A Vindication of the Rights of Whores, Angry Women, Ritual Sex *and* Living with Contradictions.

As a model, Annie has appeared in every major and minor sex magazine. Her photography has been published in American Photographer, Newsweek, Spin, Camera Austria *and* Penthouse, *and has been shown in galleries internationally. Her one-woman show, Annie Sprinkle's* Herstory of Porn – Real to Real, *is a play/film diary about her own and society's evolution through the sexual revolution. She is an excellent macrobiotic cook, loves to swim, do housekeeping, whale watch and take long nature walks. She has travelled the world extensively. Her motto is 'Let there be pleasure on earth, and let it begin with me'.*

I feel I have much more awareness around sexuality now than ever before. I am much more sensitive. I have had a very wide variety of experiences, I used to get out there and try everything and everybody, use lots of costumes, sex toys, try all kinds of fetishes and fantasies. Now I have come back to basics. I am more in tune with the spiritual side of sex, the healing aspects and exchange of the subtle energies – quiet, simple sex, but at the same time very powerful.

One thing that really turns me on lately is being out in nature. It is so sensuous, especially the ocean. I love going out on my rowboat. It's total bliss and happiness. I love the tides, and the constant change that takes place on the water. Our sexualities are so much like the ocean – always changing, fluid, sometimes calm, sometimes stormy. Sometimes it's high tide, sometimes low. I am not very promiscuous any more. I like being in very intimate relationships. I like the intimacy that comes with time. I also love to meditate and masturbate at the same time. To medibate! To allow myself to let go into the depths of erotic relaxation.

I have devoted a lot of my life to learning the art of making love. I see it a lot like painting. Each lovemaking session is a work of art! The skills of lovemaking can be learned, just like painting can be learned. I have learned a whole lot about sex from my performance work in theatre, on stage and in front of the camera. I have also explored different personas by creating different characters, wearing costumes and exploring different aspects of sex. It's been wonderful. But these days I find it important to know when 'not to perform'.

I recently attended a sex workshop taught by my friend Kutira in Germany, where we, as participants, could receive anything we wanted. Each person could ask what they needed and the whole group would help to give it to them. It could be any sort of fantasy or erotic experience. When it was my turn I asked that everyone do nothing. Everyone stood in a circle around me and did nothing for about fifteen minutes. And it was so delicious and satisfying. I got so high and turned on, and felt so much peace and bliss. Others were amazed at how powerful it was. It showed me that sometimes less is more.

We can be so busy doing a million different things: working, playing, exercising, socialising and making love that we forget how wonderful it is to do 'nothing' and just 'be'. One of my greatest discoveries was to find out that I can have an incredible, erotic orgasmic experience without doing anything. Just opening up to the erotic energy available from the universe, saying 'yes' to the ecstasy coming into the body. It's just a few breaths away.

In the one-woman show I did for several years, I performed a masturbation ritual. The idea was to evoke the spirit of the Ancient Sacred Prostitute. It was the last twenty minutes of the show. After I did it for about a year, I came to realise that it was not the excitement of building up to the climax, or the climax, I liked best. The most precious, delicious thing was during the afterglow when I was doing nothing – just being still was the most erotic, wonderful feeling.

Many couples often have just one night every so often to make love so they will aim to have a 'big orgasmic' passionate experience. It is not always necessary to make a big shebang out of it. Sometimes less is much more: often the 'subtle' is the most powerful.

I was often busy doing, doing, doing, performing, giving, receiving, putting costumes on, taking them off, building up passion and being busy, busy, busy, which was wonderful. But I discovered that doing nothing can be the most delicious, ecstatic, blissful, transformative and deeply satisfying erotic experience.

First of all, to be a great lover you must be able to look deeply into your lover's eyes and not be afraid of what you see. For the first ten years I was exploring sexuality I had tons of sex, but I did not really look deeply into people's eyes. Once I learned to look deeply into eyes, the sex got so much more intense. And far more intimate.

EXERCISE: THE ECSTASY OF DOING NOTHING (FOR COUPLES)

Time: One-and-a-half hours
Props: Clock with an alarm
Setting: In nature or in a room with candles, incense, aromatherapy (optional) but with no music, or very subtle soft music

The main thing is not to do anything, but with the intention of connecting deeply with yourself and your lover. It is not a good idea to do this exercise if you are very tired because if you fall sound asleep you will miss the effects. This exercise can be done naked or fully clothed. Use an alarm clock or timer to ring at 30-minute intervals.

Both partners should lie on their sides, in spoon position, with one person holding the other person. Close your eyes and relax your breathing. Allow yourself time to go inside your own body and into your own feelings. Make your focus relaxation – do not think about particular issues or plan future activities. Try not to think too much, but to stay very present with your lover. Let go of thoughts. You can coordinate your breathing by breathing together or by breathing alternatively, but don't be too rigid about it.

After the alarm or timer has rung, reset it for another 30 minutes. Take three deep big breaths and slowly turn over, reversing the position, with the person previously being held holding his or her partner.

When the alarm goes off again reset it for 30 minutes, but this time turn to your partner, lie in a relaxed position and hold one another. Look into each other's eyes. If you're not used to prolonged eye-gazing this can be a challenge. You may feel uncomfortable at first. Or you may feel fear that you don't like this person, or you may notice wrinkles or that he or she looks strange. Do not analyse these feelings, just let them pass through your mind. Look at your partner and allow yourself to experience whatever is there or not there, without holding onto anything. Hang in there. It's well worth learning to do it.

You may experience a trance-like feeling. You most likely will go into an altered state, and feel like you are vibrating, or floating, or very light. You may sense a metallic feeling on your tongue. You may even hallucinate a little. You may feel like you've become one and don't know where your body starts and your lover's begins. Just go with the feelings. It's all very safe. In fact, it's good for you, better than a trip to a tropical island. The experience of being held can be so beautiful. It is a very primal experience and wonderful way to express our love. When this final 30 minutes has finished give each other a passionate kiss and take a few deep breaths. If it seems hard to talk, then don't. Or if you're anxious to talk, then do. You may want to share some thoughts or feelings with each other. This exercise can create some wonderful pillow talk.

Although this sounds simple, even boring, don't knock it till you try it! You might find this is some of the best lovemaking you've ever had. It can be deeply fulfilling. Your various energy bodies are merging. Your angels might be hovering above you, enrapturing each other. You could have astral sex. What couples can learn most from this exercise is the art of being together without having to sexually perform, and you will be practising how to totally relax during lovemaking. If you do not have one-and-a-half hours do this exercise in whatever time you have, just cut the time down proportionately, say in 20-minute or 10-minute sections.

EXERCISE: THE ECSTASY OF DOING NOTHING (FOR SINGLES)

Time: 30 minutes
Props: Full-length mirror, clock with an alarm
Setting: In a room with candles, incense, aromatherapy but with no or very soft music

Set the alarm or timer for 30 minutes. Take off your clothes and, using cushions, prop up the mirror and place it in front of you so you can lie facing it on your side. Look at yourself as if you are looking at someone else. See yourself as your lover. This is a very powerful exercise because by allowing yourself to just be with yourself, by looking into your own eyes, you can create a unique intimacy with yourself. Get to know yourself better. It's fantastic.

LINDA MONTANO

This time before we are no longer fertile

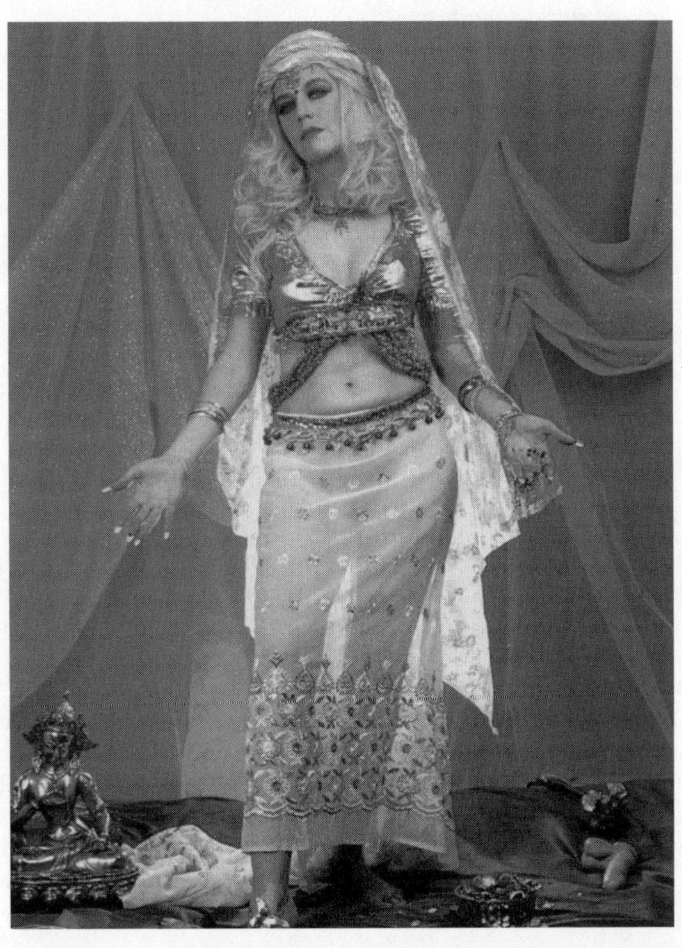

From Annie Sprinkle, *Post-Porn Modernist*

Linda Montano is a performance artist who addresses issues of endurance, life as art, art as life, humour as healing in art and life, and art as 'great therapy'. She has been performing her fears, fantasies, taboos, dreams and life issues since 1969 when she presented a performance art piece titled 'Chickens as Art' at the University of Wisconsin, Madison. In this performance, she dressed up as a dead chicken, complete with 12-foot wingspan and tap shoes.

Linda was raised a Roman Catholic and even entered the convent for two years. Since 1961 she has been addressing questions of spirituality, feminism and art, which led to research on Eastern spirituality and an experience of the rich yoga traditions of chakras, Tantra and spiritual ecstasy.

Linda translated these teachings as suggested by her meditation teacher and mentor, Dr R. S. Mishra (Brahmananda Saraswati) and has performed a fourteen-year experience from 1984 to 1998 based on the seven chakras, or energy centres. She did this by wearing clothing of only one colour, which corresponded to a particular chakra, for a twelve-month period. Each year she changed to a new colour based on the next chakra. When she completed all seven chakras, she began the cycle again. She has also performed Chakraphonics for fourteen years, a sound-based work based on a response to the energies found in the seven chakras.

While many sexuality performance artists cite Annie Sprinkle as their formative influence, Sprinkle herself acknowledges that it was Linda Montano who convinced her that she was an artist, not just a sex worker. Linda lives her art, so her personal expression is difficult to translate into tips or exercises and instead reflects her internal journey.

My most transformative sexual event occurred just before menopause, when a very strong sexual energy flooded my being. It was primal, feral, a last gasp indicating that I had hours to mate before I would no longer be able to bring a baby into the world. It was without reason and I was led by the first desire. I had no control, no sense of consequences.

Later I read that this is quite common and that this is a very powerful time for women – this time before we are no longer fertile. Women at this time are driven to procreate. I was mad with passion, insane. Out of my mind. Willing to die. And I almost did die. I was driven to the edge of madness. So my advice is to all women not yet pre-menopausal, listen when you get there and remember that every action has consequences.

TIPS FOR THE PRE-MENOPAUSAL WOMAN

• When you are about seven years from menopause, or peri-menopausal, in your late thirties or early forties, note the change in your sexual energy.

• If you are totally, wildly, passionately obsessed with someone who is not available to you, be aware of the feeling.

• Check yourself every time you want to think that you are able to do anything you want, with whomever you want, or whenever you want, even though it is not an accurate assessment of the situation.

• Write down ways that you can use your tornado of erotic energy in more beneficial ways for you and the world.

• Choose one of the suggestions and either think about that or do it.

• Thank yourself for not messing around with someone else's space, or life or wife, or husband or career or karma.

• Reward yourself.

ELIZABETH BURTON

Stripping: a creative fantasy world

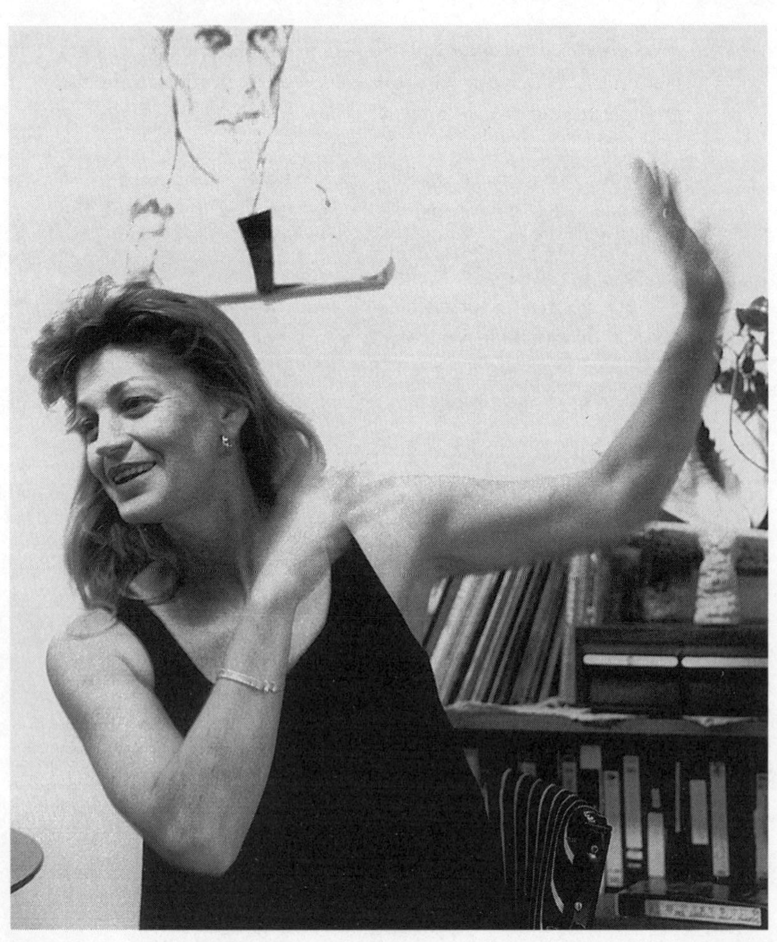

Elizabeth Burton was brought up Catholic in a tiny mining town in New South Wales, Australia. At fourteen she moved to Sydney with her family and became an apprentice hairdresser. One night a girl-friend who was a go-go dancer persuaded her to stand in for her at work as she had a double booking. Elizabeth wore an exotic costume, adlibbed some dance movements and when she heard the applause knew that she had found her calling.

She spent the next decade travelling the world – entertaining troops in Vietnam, performing throughout America and Europe in nightclubs, cabarets and appearing on film.

For many years Elizabeth taught housewives, corporate women and grandmothers how to get the most out of stripping. She is presently studying fine arts and upon graduation will become an art teacher. She has a teenage daughter.

When I first started stripping, I saw other girls being quite vulgar and decided then that if I was going to be a stripper I would present myself in the most beautiful way possible. Converting to Buddhism in 1971 helped me to achieve this in my work. According to the teaching of Buddha, the body is the temple and our instrument, and when I speak with it, this becomes my own offering and prayer.

Stripping is a dying art, which is very sad. In the days of burlesque, women appeared as part of a creative fantasy world, wearing costumes and doing elaborate routines. This has all changed – strippers today are struggling to find work. Table-top or lap dancers have taken over and there are no classy strip venues, and high-class entrepreneurs no longer pay the artists. My way of striptease was to have lots of emphasis on the tease and to wear many layers for the strip.

I have been teaching stripping to women of all ages and backgrounds for their personal development for a number of years and this has made me confident in my belief that we are all goddesses. Our body is our home, transportation, temple and place of our sexuality. My philosophy is mastication, masturbation, meditation and mobility – if we did these four things all lives would be more peaceful on earth.

No matter what shape or size you are you are perfect for you. Musically you can strip to anything, but my favourites are Joe Cocker's 'Leave Your Hat On', Larry Adler's 'The Glory of Gershwin', the soundtrack to *The Low Down Dirty Shame*, and anything by Aretha Franklin or Marvin Gaye. To do a successful strip start by creating a sexy ambience with low lighting. You can strip out of anything – from a corporate suit, casual clothes to your best dress. The more layers and props you have, the better – use gloves, layers of underwear, a hat, a feather boa, a fan.

Use a shawl to drape, tie or hold around your body for any moments of vulnerability. If you are wearing tights or stockings, roll them down your body seductively. You can even use a vibrator or sex toys in your act. Make sure your audience helps you remove your clothes. Have eye contact and a sense of humour by smiling and laughing.

Practise in a mirror the moves you wish to incorporate in your routine by holding and rotating your pelvis and becoming confident with what you wish to re-create in your dance. The routine is only limited by your imagination. To give your legs a beautiful line always point your toes. Practise walking in proper-fitting high heels, the higher the better, as this gives a very sexy look.

EXERCISE: A GUIDE TO HELP YOU WITH YOUR STRIPPING ROUTINE

- Start by standing, one foot in front of the other, stroking your body, starting from your ankle and working up the body and stretching your hands above your head.
- Posture is important: standing up straight enables you to breathe deeply and enhances your presence. When you stand up straight squeeze your bottom, lift your ribcage and relax your shoulders.
- Next, place your hands on your bottom with your knees relaxed, and do a bounce from side to side.
- To do 'the Titty Dance' grip your left wrist with your right hand and vice-versa. Push back and forward toward the elbows? This will move your pectoral muscles and make your breasts bounce.
- Throw your hands out to the side and shake your shoulders, step to the side, move your hips from side to side in time to the music. Bend your knees, rotating your hips to the right and left.
- In 'the big old booty roll' place your hand on your bent knees, stick out your bottom and rotate, screaming with delight as you do so.

Strutting. Take a big breath, stand up straight, lead with your breasts (knowing you are a goddess) and do a walk for eight counts. Freeze in a seductive pose for eight counts and repeat.

• Place your right foot in front and rotate your hips. Bend your knees and sit on the floor then lie on your back, supporting yourself with your elbows. Bend one leg and keep the other one straight. Point your toes in the air and move up and down, kicking from the knee.

• To do 'the spread', lie flat on your back, legs apart, point your toes in the air and blow kisses between your opened legs to the audience.

• Bring your legs together, recover to a sitting position with one leg over the other and stroke from the ankle all the way up the body along the side cupping your breast, running your hands up your face.

• Self-love. Roll onto your tummy, supported by your elbows and kick your legs with your knees bent. Push up to a sitting position on your knees, stroking your entire body including your genitals. Finish by bringing yourself to a standing position, one foot at a time.

• Between any of these moves you can take garments off and have the audience assist you. If you follow your piece of music it will help you time your moves.

As women started using dance and nudity to express themselves, the distinctions between the erotic, artistic and pornographic became more obvious. Dance and nudity have gone on to be used by feminists to celebrate the female body, protest against the restrictions put upon it by society and reclaim their sexuality without being seen as simply lewd.

In 1975 in the US Carolee Schneeman in a performance entitled 'Interior Scroll' pulled a dream written on a scroll from her vagina, daring to offer the public her interior life and vision. She challenged the distinction between art, life, the body and pornography and she has inspired women performance artists in the decades since. Other artists, such as international model Verushka, used their body as a canvas on which artists could create a human artwork.

A backlash occurred within the ranks of feminism by the early 1980s. Many women campaigning against sexual violence saw sexual performance artists as part of the adult industry that they believed perpetuated attitudes that caused violence against women. In this way female sexual performance artists, and certainly women who worked in the sex industry, were regarded as guilty by association. Feminism was split and the consequences of the so-called 'sex wars' of the 1980s still reverberate today. The women who became the sexual radicals of the 1980s believed that the way they expressed their bodies and their sexuality was fluid. They saw that women could control their own destiny to find pleasure, replacing the feminism of the 1970s, seen by some as relying on domination, fear and alienating women from their own bodies. This led to women who were sex performers.

Women who were sex performers and feminist sex workers joined forces and declared themselves feminists and pro-sex activists, later describing themselves as 'sex positivists'. They also started to organise within the adult industry to have more control over their work and the representation of female sexuality. They used their political consciousness to campaign for better wages and conditions. In this they followed in the tradition of Gypsy Rose Lee who organised a union for burlesque artists in 1951. (Until the 1980s peep shows artists were frequently not paid a wage and their only income came from tips.)Performance artists such as Annie Sprinkle draw on her work in the sex industry to make a new kind of body-orientated performance art. Annie made her solo debut as a performance artist in 1985. She performed throughout the US and Europe and found people who were fascinated by her insight into the sex industry and how she used her body. Increasingly women in the adult industry crossed over into formerly 'artistic' performance work and staked their claim to be considered legitimate artists. In doing so the power dynamic between the artist and the audience changed.

From an almost all-male audience for their adult shows, these artists now had a new following of feminists, bohemians and the inner-city trendy. Their work was no longer viewed as just explicit, but as 'experimental' and 'cutting edge'. A female audience brought a different perspective to their work and it changed and developed under the female gaze. They no longer played with pleasing men, but instead pleased themselves.

2

Spiritual Sexuality

Spiritual sexuality is the buzzword of the new millennium and has become synonymous with techniques based on ancient Indian and Chinese teachings. The word '*tantra*' is Hindu Sanskrit in origin and means 'to extend, expand and weave'. Therefore Tantric sex is a process of interconnectedness between ourselves and the universe, as well as an internal expansion into pleasure.

The Chinese word '*tao*' means 'communion with the Universe' and the harmony between *yin* (night/female) and *yang* (day/male), and the energy between the two. Both philosophies expand into lovemaking, with the weaving of energies internally and externally with a partner. A 'Tantrica' or 'taoist' is someone who has taken these philosophies as the basis of experiencing their life.

In the West we assume that we jump into bed with someone and a deep sense of connection will automatically happen. Traditional tantricas, on the other hand, practise techniques of breath, movement and visualisation for months, even years, before they would make love to a partner.

Sex becomes 'spiritual' when it moves away from a focus on genital orgasms, and can be felt as more of a heart-genital connection. Then it becomes something you can take outside of yourself to connect with another or the universe. Meditation through breathing, movement or light can be fused with sexual energy and this can lead to deep erotic experiences. The beauty of experiencing a deeper level of sexuality and spirituality is not limited by your relationship status, sexual preference or age.

Chakras are the energy centres of the body and located from the perineum to the top of the head. This concept is Indian in origin and explains the flow of energy throughout the body. It became popular in the West in the 1960s, when meditation and yoga found a new mainstream audience. Knowledge of the chakras can be used to open up the senses and expand your concept of sexual pleasure. There are seven chakras, each associated with a specific colour and a sense.

- The first chakra is at the perineum, which is between the anus and the genitals and is associated with the colour red, your sense of smell, the urge to survive and your fight or flight response.
- The second is at the genitals and associated with your sense of

taste, the colour orange and your sexual energy.

•The third is just above the navel and is associated with the colour yellow, the adrenals, pancreas, digestive organs and the emotions anger, fear and jealousy.

•The fourth chakra is at the heart, in the middle of the chest and is associated with the colour green, the sense of touch, thymus gland and emotions of love and compassion.

•The fifth is at the base of the throat and associated with the colour blue, the thyroid gland, sense of hearing and relates to creativity and verbal expression.

•The sixth chakra is located between and slightly above your eyebrows and is known as 'the third eye'. Its colour is indigo and is the centre for intuition and wisdom. It is related to the sense of sight and the pineal gland.

•The seventh chakra is located at the top of your head, the colour is violet and is the point of illumination and spirituality.

•There are also chakras located in the palms of your hands associated with giving and receiving and the souls of the feet to feel connected to the earth.

There are many forms of orgasms and orgasmic experiences associated with spiritual sexuality, but the one most sought after is the full body orgasm. In this sexual pleasure is experienced as waves of energy pulsing throughout the body and can be felt for seconds, minutes or even hours. Once you have learned full-body orgasm techniques by yourself, then it is easier to experience this with another.

During a full-body orgasm some people experience a feeling of warmth or tingling throughout their body and the feeling of having their system either cleaned out or highly invigorated. Other people see light or specific colours in their chakras and especially in the heart, throat, third eye and crown. The emphasis in a full-body orgasm is to move the energy created in the genitals up and throughout the body. Wilheim Reich's research on the orgasmic response focused on four stages: tension, charge, release and relaxation.

Spiritual sexuality is about expanding the charge in the body for hours instead of minutes before the release or orgasm. Men are taught how to orgasm, but not ejaculate, which in the West is usually synonymous. In tantric and taoist practices these are two separate physical experiences, and men can learn to control ejaculation, to extend the period of lovemaking, and not to rapidly dissipate their erotic energy. They then learn to be in control of the sexual sensations in their body, rather than the reverse. For women the main focus in spiritual sexuality is the spread of orgasmic energy throughout the body, which can be done with or without a physical orgasm.

In my private practice much of my work is based on teaching people how to expand their body sensations by learning specific tantric breathing and moving techniques. When you deepen your own body's sensations you realise that you do not have to find the perfect partner in order to change your sensual and erotic experience of life. If a partner comes it is a blessing, but it is not a prerequisite for pleasure. My clients have told me that when they experience more aliveness in their body, their senses expand proportionately and they feel more connected to the people around them and life itself.

In this chapter the wisdom of Jwala, Kutira and Cora, who collectively have spent decades exploring spiritual sexuality, will uplift and inspire you.

CORA EMENS

Your Body as your temple of Love

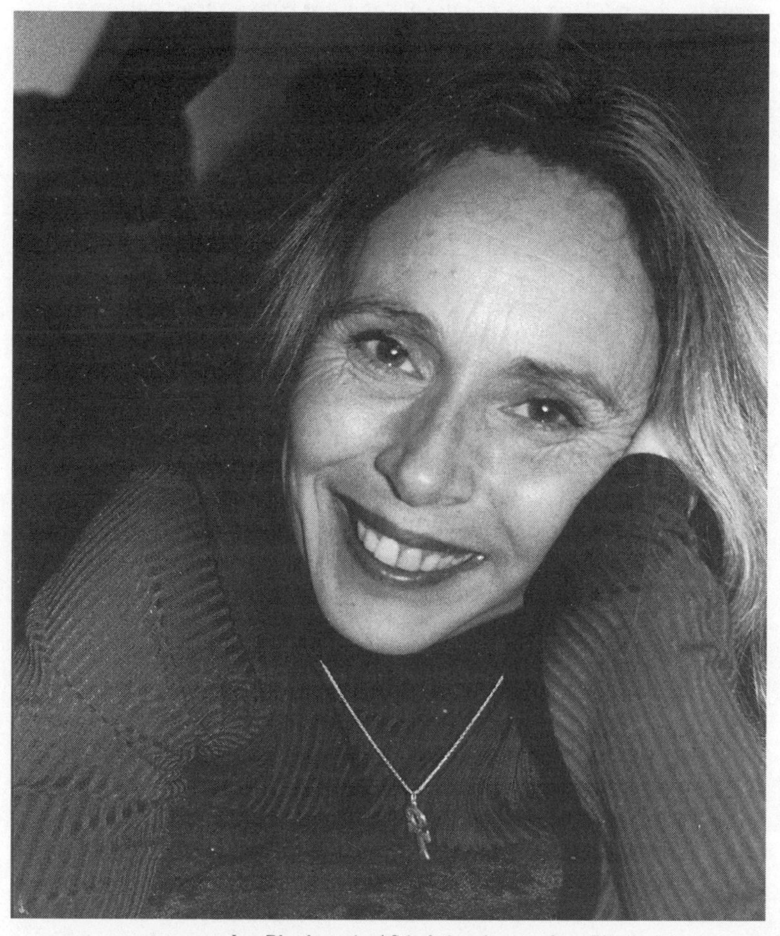

Jan Blankestein / Stitchting Amsterdam Photo Art

Cora Emens was born in the Netherlands and studied to be a health teacher, but decided to devote her energies to improving the sex and sexual status of other women. She has studied and assisted in self-loving (masturbation) workshops conducted by Joseph Kramer and Dr Betty Dodson in the US, and has participated in the seminars and performance art of her best friends Annie Sprinkle and Willem de Ridder in North America and Europe. In 1990 she became the first person to organise and lead self-loving workshops for women in the Netherlands as well as erotic massage courses for couples.

Cora is a nationally recognised spokesperson for women's sexual rights, with her own weekly radio show, which has broken rating records. After television appearances Cora Emens was besieged with thousands of letters requesting a more detailed or personal instruction in the art of sexual gratification. To answer these she made a video showing a group of women who are learning how to love themselves and how to masturbate.

She has created, with her life partner Shai Shahar, the website www.sex4life. They are also proud parents of two 13-year-old daughters. It is to them, and the sons and daughters of the next millennium, that they dedicate their work.

The key to making sex a spiritual experience is totally in the eye of the beholder. In this case I would say in the eyes of the person(s) having it. And that is all that matters. The way to attain such an experience does not matter at all. But the experience has such a profound impact once we do, that all we want is to repeat it. So, naturally, being human led us to inventing ways to 'get there'. Or maybe we were taught by 'higher beings', only God knows.

We can find reflections of the 'way(s)' in the teachings and practices in ancient temples and in sacred places. Today you can buy books and videos everywhere to learn 'how to have spiritual sex'. Having a spiritual experience teaches us about death and sex launches us right into that – 'the little death'. Through a sexual, spiritual experience we consciously experience how closely related life and death are.

And right there we discover 'Self', that it is all about the Self, that even the Other is the Self, only projected outward. Some will reach this state while 'under the influence' of sex with stimulants and/or through intensive dancing, like old shamans in new bodies. Others may reach it through the disciplined practice of certain (yoga) positions or breathing patterns. Yet others don't seem to need any kind of preparation at all. It is natural for them.

I believe that it is possible for anybody who wills it to have sex as a spiritual experience at any time, even when the partner is not 'spiritual' at all. The big question is, do you want sex to be a spiritual experience? And if you do, are you willing to totally experience sex as an earthy, lusty experience? Are you willing to accept your body as your temple of lust? The 'lust for life' is the source of all creation. Are you willing to experience that lust running like fire through your body, heightening your senses, accelerating the speed of your vibration, sweeping away your ego? Are you willing to learn to stay in touch with the Self while all this lovely madness is going on within you? Are you willing to be confronted with your wounds, scars and flaws? Question your learned belief-systems and responses? Find and accept your true Self whether you have a lover or not? You will find a master key there, which will fit any other true heart.

A Masturbation Ritual to Get What You Want

I have always looked at sex as something sacred, something really important that 'they' did not have the right to take away from me. It was the key to myself. Through sex I could get in contact with another world that I recognised as 'home'. I was so happy with this new connection – I could actually touch a button on my body that suddenly took me someplace else! To me, masturbation was a reunion of energies. Suddenly I had access to a world I did not fully understand yet, and it was one of pretty high vibrations. Masturbating for me meant learning to play with these higher vibrations.

My body would tell me exactly how far to go in containing so much energy and an orgasm would release me from too much so it would not be dangerous to my system. I am still happy I gave myself this training despite the hostility against sex in my parents' house.

But I have my load of guilt and it took me a long time to get rid of most of that – the remainder I have learned how to play with. So I started out really young but lost most of my awareness as I grew up.

Still, masturbation has always been important to me and I even made a profession out of it by teaching masturbation courses. I keep on finding out things about myself, so for me, my self-loving-sessions can be transformative.

Because I really take the time for such sessions, which include dancing or a nice relaxing shower, I can sink into a kind of 'transformed state of being' and that makes me more receptive for self-contemplation, while being sexual. Do not get me wrong, I do like to share this with my partner, but sometimes it just concerns me and I do not need him to masturbate with, although that can be fun too.

Before I met my partner I had one of these sessions I masturbated myself up to a very high vibrational state, building the picture in my head of my 'perfect' lover and partner in life. And he was (is!) a really beautiful man. Handsome too: high cheekbones, some royal features, a charming smile, loving but straight eyes – what else could I go for? But more than that, a real man. In my masturbation ritual I let myself roam in my feelings of lust and what I would like him to do. Which secret he would know about me instantly. I wanted him to be dominant, to know about my tits, my fire, my capacity, my impatience. Sexually he would play with me, but I want to make peace and give myself over to that man on the moment I'd come because I would love him. He was the man I wanted, and wanted to share this with. All my energy was directed outward in one big blast. I came, and all of me cried out in silence, 'yes!'.

I met him within fourteen days. I recognised him immediately and we have a very strong connection, spiritually as well as sexually. We live together with our two daughters. We are all happy to have found each other. The spiritual/sexual experience of masturbation changed my whole life. I recommend that you do not try this at home without practice – lots of practice!

JWALA

Breathing opens up a sense of pleasure

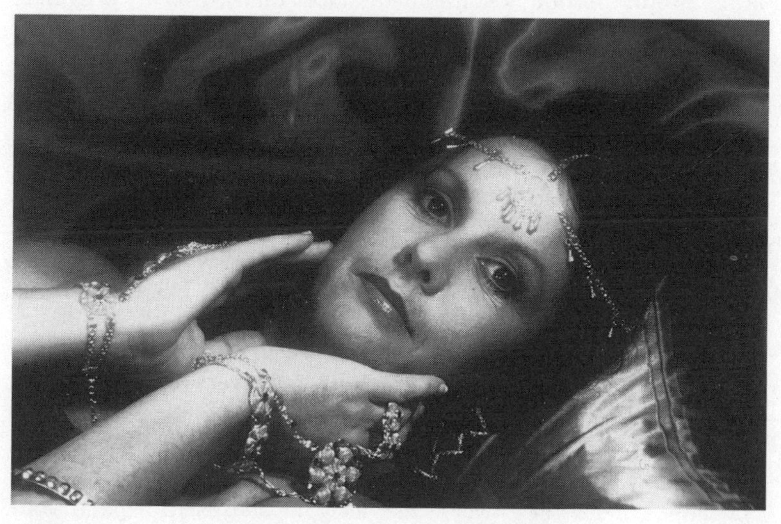

Jwala, whose name means 'volcanic fire', has taught Tantra in the US, India, Italy, England and Australia for the past twenty-one years. She was born in the US, but has travelled the world and now calls San Francisco home. In her workshops and individual sessions she teaches participants to make lovemaking a sacred experience. Her book Sacred Sex explores positions, breathing techniques and rituals which are the foundations of her work. She began Tantric studies in 1969 with a couple and became an apprentice in 1970. Her teachers include Osho (Rajneesh), Sunyati Saraswati, Leonard Orr and Harley Swift Deer.

Jwala's work has transformed many people's sex lives and her talents include interior and costume design for theatre, film and everyday life. Her company, Goddess for Hire, provides a wide range of unique and unusual services from redesigning lovemaking areas into interior erotic environments to Tantra-grams, providing entertainment with sensual dancers, love teams, rituals and party events. She has produced her own video Ecstatica and appears in the video *The Tantric Journey to Female Orgasm*.

Even though sensuality and the art of sensuality has been a continual thread my whole adult life, I am now looking at my passion in a new way. What is happening now, during menopause, is that my sexuality and sensuality are now directed inwards. It is a very different experience for me; sex is very intense but it is not as frequent.

Ritual and focusing on conscious breathing have opened the door on my personal path. If I could only tell lovers one thing in bed it would be to breathe, and to make sure they did not ever hold their breath, even in excitement. Breathing opens up a sense of pleasure and prolongs orgasm. Imagine that you were looking at, and smelling, a beautiful flower – use all your senses to expand your sense of pleasure.

What I do as a Tantrica is to initiate people into the arts of Tantra through workshops, classes, celebrations, ceremonies and individual or couple's sessions. As a teacher of ancient sexual secrets, I am a catalyst to inspire the unaware to go for more liveliness and juicyness. By continuing to strive to become a more spiritually and sexually enlightened woman, I may serve as a role model for others. When people are turned on, their joy is infectious.

There are a number of key things you can include in your

lovemaking, with yourself or with another, that will make sex a more spiritual experience. First choose a time when you and your partner are relaxed and not rushed, and a place where you feel safe. Speak the truth of what you need and what you want every time you make love. If you want something different, learn to be able to say it to your partner without fear.

If you are setting up the following ritual, start by communicating. I now take this into lovemaking as I have no hesitation to say to a partner 'let's try this position', or to say 'breathe' if I notice he or she is not breathing. I want to debunk the myth that speaking during lovemaking is not romantic. I have watched the whole direction of lovemaking change by being willing to say 'if you touch my clitoris a little higher, I would feel five times more erotic'.

Part of this is learning how to say things in a way that makes your partner feel loved and appreciated. It is important to acknowledge the person verbally by saying 'I love your touch and what I would like now is [insert what you would like] as this would give me more pleasure'. When your lover does this acknowledge it, 'Oh yes, like that'. This is very helpful, and allows you and your partner to communicate during lovemaking. We limit ourselves when we allow our erotic map, that is, our past sexual experiences, to be the only way we can expand our erotic pleasure.

EXERCISE: TANTRA RITUAL FOR EROTIC SENSUALITY

I have been using a set ritual for twenty-eight years, which has become a basis for myself and the people I have taught to go to a very deep level of emotional and sexual intimacy.

Adorn the room or the sexual space with beautiful flowers, massage oil and candles. Remember that in creating an erotic environment, draw on the four elements – fire, earth, air and water – to make your lovemaking a total bodily experience. Fire can be expressed by lighting candles, or if you have a fireplace in your room focus on the flames and take this feeling within yourself and into your lovemaking.

The earth element can be expressed by fruits, which can be cut up and used as taste treats on your partner's body.

Air is felt through our conscious breathing patterns, and the more we breathe the more energy we feel and integrate into our body.

The water element is internalised by drinking glasses of liquid, be they water or juice.

We often see orgasm as the peak erotic experience, after which we cannot go on any further. Tantra is about learning to tolerate higher degrees of sexual energy and breathing will allow the spread of this energy around the body. You can even take this orgasmic energy into meditation. By going to different experimental heights you can move from being passionate, to meditative and then back again. When you take the energy to that level it is very different from the first biological sexual release. I acknowledge it in the body and also outside in the physical space we are using.

It is important to open up the sense organs and then the chakras or energy centres, so that by the time I get into lovemaking my sensuality is turned on and the cultivated passion can travel throughout the body. I start to open up the senses as they are connected to the chakras and opening them up allows more pleasure to be felt.

Glasses of fluids represent the elements – springwater; fire element would be alcohol or spirits, for example a glass of wine; earth element would be a glass of exotic fruit juice such as pineapple or a coconut drink. Air element would be to control the temperature with a fan or heater.

Bathing ritual

Create a sensual space in the bathroom with candles, scents, aromatherapy or incense, place grapes in the bathtub and have a glass of fruit juice available. Lie in the bath by yourself for about seven minutes then invite your partner in and play for seven minutes, then get out of the bath and allow your partner seven minutes to relax alone. Do not stay in the bath longer because it will drain your energy, which is needed for lovemaking.

If you don't have a bath use a large bowl of hot water and use a wash cloth to wash one another. To be washed is a very beautiful nurturing experience. Hand-washing rituals can also be done using flowers or rosewater in a bowl.

Clearing on the mental plane

Release anything that is blocking you. This can also include safe sex practices, how far the two of you can go and feel safe with one another. Each partner says, 'Do you have any withheld communication from me?' Praise and spend time appreciating one another. Acknowledge your partner, 'Oh you look lovely tonight, I really like how you have put special attention into adorning yourself.

Communication without words
Sit opposite one another, place your right hand in between your partner's chest or heart chakra, and your left hand on the hand that is on your chest or heart chakra. Take a few deep breaths through your mouth and allow your eyes to connect with your partner's, which opens up the 'love centre'. This is very healing and centring and allows you to express any emotion, be it sadness or joy, and is a way of connecting your lower three chakras with your upper three chakras.

EXERCISE: KUNDALINI MEDITATION

The day before I meet my lover I always do a Kundalini meditation to release my bodily tension and prepare myself. This meditation makes a big difference to lovemaking because it opens up the body.

Time: 1 hour divided into four 15-minute parts
Music: For parts 1 and 2, something with a definite beat, such as dance, African or world music. For parts 3 and 4, no music

Part 1 (15 minutes): With your eyes closed stand in the one spot with your knees bent. Start to shake your whole body, letting go of any tension or frustration you are feeling.
Part 2 (15 minutes): With your eyes open or closed, dance, allowing your body to move to the rhythm.
Part 3 (15 minutes): This part is to bring meditation into play. You sit and remain silent, watching the mind, becoming a witness as if your thoughts were on a movie screen.
Part 4 (15 minutes): Lie down and feel the support of the ground beneath you, helping you relax.

KUTIRA

The orgasm is with the universe

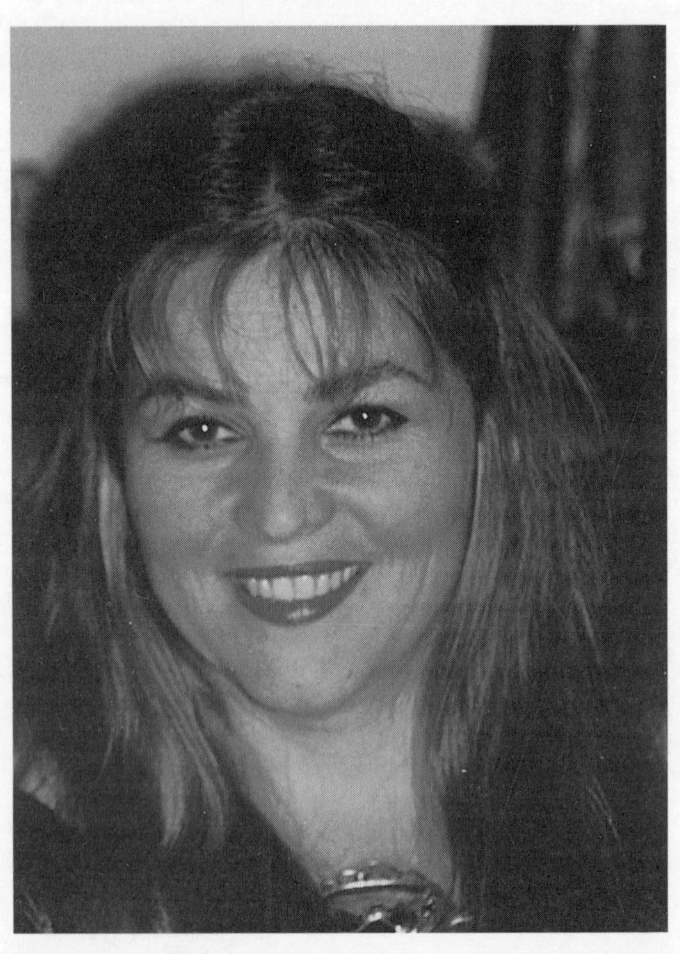

Kutira Decosterd was born and raised in Switzerland. She lived in India for two years, studying with Tantric masters from the East and West. She also has a strong background in meditation, breath work, neuro-linguistic programming, Hokomi (body-centred psychotherapy), bioenergetics, Gestalt, movement therapy, communications, sexual therapy and massage.

Kutira, whose name means 'Temple of Love', is an internationally acknowledged Tantra teacher, creator of Oceanic Tantra and the founder of the Kahua Hawaiian Institute. She gracefully combines ancient Tantric and Taoist practices of energy-raising, music, yoga, psychology, marine ecology and meditation with a planetary vision and dolphin consciousness. During the winter months in Hawaii, Kutira conducts Whale Adventures in Consciousness with Dr John C. Lilly, one of the twentieth-century's foremost scientific pioneers of the inner and outer limits of human experience.

Kutira and her partner Raphael have been in a loving Tantric marriage for many years. Much of their Tantra philosophy has been practised and perfected in this period, which they share in their seminars.

Together Kutira and Raphael have released eleven music albums, including Music to Disappear in I and II, Tantric Wave *and* Intimacy, *and a video,* Surrender to Love. *They live together in Maui, Hawaii, and are directors of the Kahua Hawaiian Institute. Their work has been featured on a number of American and European television networks, as well as in many international magazines. Twice a year they teach a retreat on Maui and present seminars or rituals and concerts in the US and Europe. They also make themselves available for private couples' retreats, Tantric weddings and other healing sessions.*

Growing up in a Judaeo Christian tradition doesn't leave you much space to embrace sexuality with spirituality. After I finished my studies in Switzerland, I was fortunate to travel to other countries such as India and Nepal. It was in India that I first saw, in a temple, that sexuality can be honoured within the spiritual path. It took me a while to reframe my belief systems about sexuality. In the temple, on the altar, I saw a *lingam* (which represents the male sexual organ) joined in a *yoni* (which represents the female sexual organ) as a sacred aspect of the union of man and woman.

It was worshipped and celebrated, which for me opened up other doors of understanding sexuality within a spiritual context.

Regardless of how spiritual your focus in this lifetime becomes, until you acknowledge that you are a sexual being, until you awaken and align all of your chakras, you cannot experience a state of completeness, wholeness and balance.

In the 1970s, while travelling in India, I came across the Master Bhagwan Shree Rajneesh (now called Osho), who spoke of the state of orgasm being the closest thing most humans know to the state of bliss and dissolving into a state of no-mind, peace, love and happiness. I became a follower of Osho, which allowed me to explore sexuality in its fullest potential. The master gave me a name that put me into learning to accept the body as an instrument of god/goddess. The name Ma Prem Kutira (which means 'Temple of Love') was not what I expected or wanted. I was expecting a more 'spiritual' name. I asked myself, simply 'a temple', a constructed booth? I was expecting and wanted a name that was more enlightened. Temple of Love? I had to learn to understand that our body is the instrument of pleasure and spiritual grounding, which is basically love, but love for the universe. If you fine-tune your temple, accept and love your temple, greater pleasures and higher states of being are possible. Now after all these years, my body is viewed as a divine temple that holds the sacredness.

Some of the names that we give our bodies show how deeply we are in denial of the sacred parts. For example, in German, pubic hair is called *schamhaare*, hair of shame. What does that tell you? Touching the hair of shame. What shame? Where do we go with messages like that? Our language has given some rather bad names to the most sacred places of our bodies, of our temples. In the English language, they use words like dick, willy, pussy, cunt. It's a turn-off, as in something degrading. We can call them by more beautiful names, like *lingam*, lightning wand or *yoni*, crystal cave.

These places need to be honoured and touched as much as other parts of your body, but if you approach them from a degrading aspect it comes from greed, horniness or lust. If you touch them as the creative mothering or fathering aspect of the body, honour them as sacred pathways of pleasure and love and spiritual union, then you touch them with reverence. These are key things which are necessary to include with yourself or your partner to make sex a spiritual experience.

Tantra is an ancient mystical path that offers an all-embracing vision of cosmic harmony. Tantra involves the expansion of liberation of consciousness, making it the fabric of life. The key thing is the heart, the feelings, being penetrated into your soul. With yourself, that means loving yourself, loving your body and accepting yourself in its fullest. How can you love another without loving yourself? With a partner, it means opening yourself up to your partner from your heart and nowhere else, not from your *yoni*, not from his *lingam*.

Your focus is to get into the heart and come from love, and no technique is as powerful as that simple and primary beginning place. Surrender is the key to ecstasy. To allow intimacy and to know that when you look into your partner's eyes, you're looking into your partner's soul. That makes the spiritual experience.

When you ask yourself when you had the best sex, wasn't it when it penetrated your heart, when your minds merged into one, when there were tears in your eyes? In Tantra, the orgasm is with the universe. All that leads into the orgasm is physical, but the orgasm itself is a spiritual experience. There is no sense of yesterday, no tomorrow, only the here and now, this very moment.

In French, they call it *la petite mort*, the little death. An orgasm is like a little death, a surrender into the *mahamudra*, the great orgasm with the universe. When you and your partner are attuned and you connect on every level, body, mind, heart and soul you truly travel into dimensions of greater consciousness.

EXERCISE: OCEANIC TANTRA RITUAL

You can do this exercise alone or with your partner. Dolphins and whales are a source of inspiration and an important bridge to Tantra. Their conscious breathing and undulatory movements are similar to the breathing and movement techniques taught in traditional Tantric practices. These practices move the cerebral-spinal fluid and the Kundalini force (the body's biological life energy system) from the base of the spine to the brain, creating an energy frequency connection to God or Goddess, the Divine, the Force, the Oneness. When you are touched with the pulse of these energy waves, everything becomes orgasmic. You can make love to everything, let go of all barriers to pure bliss.

When, after a busy day, I want to reconnect with my husband, the fastest path to our hearts is sitting or lying together holding each other and breathing long deep breaths in matching rhythm; letting go, surrendering into the beingness within us. Our other favourite ritual that encompasses the breathing together is music. Both Raphael and I have been vitally involved in music to create the mood for intimacy and transformation. We actually met ten years ago during the time I was recording Into the Dreamtime, ritualistic music to enhance conscious breathing and the Tantric practice of 'the wave'.

First on, use some New Age music with a definite beat. Start this exercise using conscious breathing, with more emphasis on the inhale rather than the exhale. Either lie down or stand up, then move your pelvis, allowing an undulation to move throughout your body. Imagine you are a whale swimming through the limitless blue ocean. Let the pelvis move backward as you inhale; bring the pelvis forward as you exhale. Let the movement become stronger and feel the undulatory movement through your spine, including the neck.

Visualise the flow of energy rising from your first chakra along the spine, up to your crown chakra, and back to your first chakra, creating a circle of energy. The conscious breathing and the movement of the wave creates an energy frequency that opens up to the universal mind, the oneness of life. This particular practice, the Tantric Wave Ritual, helps to loosen the pelvis and brings more energy into your body.

3

Gender Bending

Many people wonder what it would be like to cross gender, to walk in the shoes of the opposite sex and experience life from 'the other side'. Men have traditionally used the excuse of a fancy dress party or a sports club social night to throw on a frock, push two balloons down the front of their dress and slip on some high heels.

Women are just as fascinated with masculinity and maleness, but rarely have the same opportunity to playfully cross-dress. Many women wonder what they can get away with if they can 'pass' off as a man and have male power and influence in the public domain, even if it was just for a day.

In the collection *Dick for a Day*, some women writers were asked what they would do if they had a penis for a day. Their answers were fascinating and frequently hilarious because they touched on women's intrigue with penis 'power'. Many women used their personal phallic experiences to try to get inside the male psyche, an area that is otherwise culturally off-limits. Almost all of them reported a feeling of power because of their new appendage.

Interestingly, this is reflected in many films, from men's experience of throwing on a frock in *Tootsie* and *Mrs Doubtfire* to women taking on a male persona in *Sylvia Scarlett* and Barbra Streisand in *Yentl*. However, men's and women's experience of publicly taking on another gender is very different. As film critic and historian Vito Russo has noted, when men dress as women they become disempowered in the social world, but when women dress as men they become empowered.

Historically, when women have cross-dressed it has been about survival. Whether they were fleeing an abusive family, a violent husband or a threatened arrest, cross-dressing and passing as a man has allowed many a woman the social freedom of movement which made escape possible. Other women have dressed as men in order to have adventurous jobs, such as being a doctor or a pilot, which would probably have been denied to them because of their gender. Others still wanted to experience the excitement of running away to sea, or off to war, and dressed as men in order to make this possible. Marjorie Garber, in her book *Vested Interests* (1992) lists many examples of women who went about for most of their lives disguised as men – from Anne Bonny and Mary Read, two eighteenth-century pirates who dressed as men, to Dr Eugene Perkins, a Californian physician who was found on 'his' death in 1936 to be a woman, and

Billy Tipton, a jazz musician, whose wife didn't even know that her husband was a woman. Even today cultural or religious restrictions on women's freedom mean that they cross-dress in order to have the same rights that men naturally enjoy.

Although most people are happy with their biological gender, many people feel androgynous, that is, like both a man and a woman. Although gender-bending is more acceptable than previously – with the androgynous look popularised by designers such as Calvin Klein and Jean-Paul Gautier prominent in glossy magazines and on the catwalk – outside this artistic world discrimination and even violence continue. This is even more shocking when what is traditionally masculine or feminine is now totally up for grabs. Sex roles and relationships have undergone enormous changes with the freeing up of restrictions based on appearances and perceived gender alone. One of the most interesting gender phenomenon of the last decade has been women's claim to inclusion in the most traditional area of cross-gender exploration – drag. Drag has traditionally been male-to-female cross-dressing, and usually the sole preserve of gay culture, which has embraced its male-female duality. In the gay communities different types of visual gender expression, such as masculine women and feminine men, are generally viewed more compassionately than in mainstream society. Given this, it is not surprising that it has been a gay and lesbian environment that has most nurtured female drag.

As women have started to 'perform' male gender, they have created their own drag king personas, many with an individual idiosyncratic style. Some drag king characters have become so well-known that they have loyal female and male followings that travel long distances to see them perform.

Many of these early drag king performers were approached by other women who wanted help in creating their own male characters. Some of the women were interested in public performance, but others simply wanted to explore the idea of getting in touch with their 'inner male'. This did not mean just getting in touch with male characteristics, such as aggression and a forceful sexuality, but also giving physical embodiment to this masculine part of their psyche. In short, if you brought out your inner male – what would he look like?For women attending drag king workshops the answers have often been surprising. Some women have discovered a sensitive New Age man lurking within, while others have given full rein to a traditional male chauvinist. Other women have had inner male characters with sexual expressions ranging from a heterosexual womaniser to a leather-clad gay man. Many women have cross-dressed only to find, often to their surprise, that their inner male is not at all what they expected.

Women get emotionally trapped when they can only see themselves in a stereotypically female way. To watch someone else break the gender barrier and step outside their role is liberating and to do it yourself is even more empowering. In a drag king workshop a woman is forced to learn to draw on her own inner resources and throw off her socially defined role as someone's wife, sister, daughter or mother.

In this chapter Veronica Vera, Shelly Mars, norrie mAy-welby and Diane Torr take on gender stereotypes and blow them wide apart. They explore what it means to act out, even live out, multiple gender identities and how this can expand your world.

VERONICA VERA

Grateful men in skirts

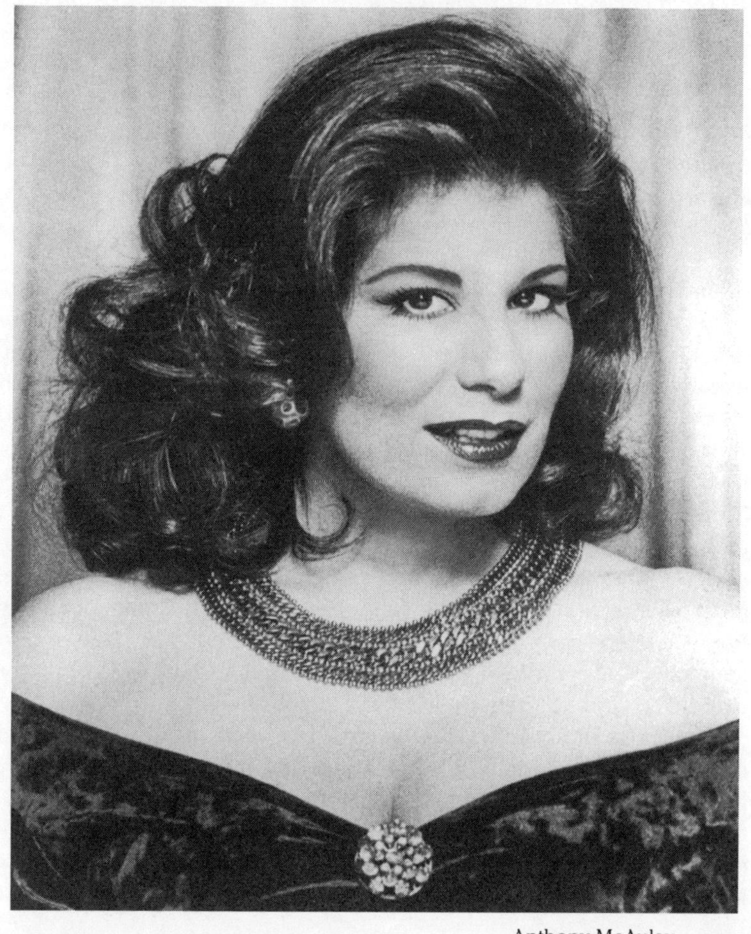

Anthony McAulay

Veronica Vera is the Dean of Miss Vera's Finishing School For Boys Who Want To Be Girls, the world's original cross-dressing academy. She started out as a stock trader on Wall Street but her religious repression inspired her to become a porn star and prolific sex writer. She has modelled for Robert Mapplethorpe and Joel-Peter Wilkin and has also been a cable TV sex-news anchorperson.

Her political career led her to become a founding member of Club 90, the world's first support group for actresses from the porn industry, and she has testified before the Meese Commission on obscenity by reading her erotic prose and showing photos of herself in bondage.

She is an activist for Prostitutes of New York (PONY) in the decriminalisation of prostitution. She is also on the board of directors of Feminists for Free Expression and has written hundreds of articles on human sexuality. Her book, Miss Vera's Finishing School For Boys Who Want To Be Girls, *is a step-by-step guide for a male-to-female transformation which provides a wonderful insight into her experiences. The following piece is derived from 'An Orientation Message From Veronica Vera, Dean of Students, Miss Vera's Finishing School For Boys Who Want To Be Girls' from the book.*

From the time I established Miss Vera's Finishing School For Boys Who Want To Be Girls in New York, my pink Princess phone began to ring incessantly. At the other end of the line were the often nervous, usually husky, sometimes breathy, mostly polite and always excited voices of the men – the Stephanies and Jennifers, Denises and JoAnns, the prospective students, all of whom wanted to explore their feminine side. They felt her like children feel an imaginary friend. Often, she had been with them since childhood. Some could look in the mirror and see her in their eyes. In learning of the academy they felt they had found someone who believed in her too. Most callers asked me if the school was for real. Could I actually help them to 'pass' as female? When I answered 'yes', it was as if someone had confirmed the existence of Santa Claus or, as I prefer to think of myself, Cinderfella's fairy godmother.

I quickly felt myself riding the crest of a wave of success, uplifted on the broad shoulders of a sea of grateful men in skirts. Not only had I put my well-manicured finger on the pulse of every cross-dresser's dream, but I had tapped into the rich motherlode of the male psyche. Having gone through my own process of woman's liberation, I understood my students as the flip side of the feminist movement. When women felt the need for balance in their lives, to share more in the male experience – to move from the home to the workplace, from the bedroom to the boardroom, to be financially independent, and sexually autonomous – we created the women's movement. Men, too, have this need for balance, to share more in what they view as the most desirable aspects of the female experience: to be pampered and protected, to be glamorous and sexually desirable, and, yes, even to do housework – many of the 'privileges' that we women saw as confining. Cross-dressers are more fortunate than most men because their affinity for the clothing gives them access to these feelings of Venus envy. The Academy offers a mode of action. For every woman who burned her bra, there is a man ready to wear one.

The Academy is my own private laboratory. With the matriculation of more than 500 on-campus students, I have been able to witness the positive aspects of this unique form of behaviour modification. Contrary to what many assume, the student is not 'finished' when he puts on a dress and learns to carry himself like a debutante, but rather when he can take the lessons and insights of his femmeself and integrate them into his male persona.

Robert is a student who came to the academy every six weeks. One of our early classes consisted of a field trip during which Robert and I visited a tiny lingerie shop in Chelsea. With the help of the shop's proprietress, we chose some frilly bra and panty sets and lacy nighties for Robert to try on in the shop's private dressing-room. Our plan was to leave the store with our purchases, to have dinner together and then return to the Academy where, with the aid of cosmetics and prosthetics, Robert would become Roberta and model her new finery. During dinner I was aghast as I watched Robert eat. He hunched over his plate and shovelled the food into his mouth.

'Roberta will need lessons in table manners,' I told him. Robert explained that his professional life as a doctor left him no time for table manners. Eating for him was just something he needed to accomplish in order to go on cutting people up. He proceeded to tell me that his schedule was overbooked, that he did not know how to say 'no' to people, and that he feared for his health as he learned of colleagues who had heart attacks at an early age. Here was a man who wanted to dress in soft delicate clothes but was still imprisoned in a tough male hide.

But clothes alone do not make the woman. As I tell every student: understand that when you dress there may be things that you also need to address. I saw very clearly that Roberta, the femmeself could, through lessons in etiquette and table manners at the Academy, learn to eat more slowly and with more appreciation for the nourishing pleasure of food, and thus lead Robert to a longer and happier life. As the butterfly Roberta emerged from her cocoon, she lessened Robert's chances of dropping like a fly. I am sure that her lessons with the knife and fork improved his skill with a scalpel.

Such success stories are the goal of Miss Vera's Finishing School. Are we encouraging a band of defectors? Undermining the male power structure? I prefer to think that we are responding to a need. The tremendous popularity of the Academy attests to the fact that people want to believe that there is a place where men can learn to be more like women. This is an idea whose time has come.

In those other academic circles, gender is a discipline; in publishing, it's a genre; in cyberspace, an option; in show business, it's a gimmick. The topic has captured the international zeitgeist. Now, more than ever, there is great awareness that gender roles are in a state of flux. All of this reflects the public's fascination and awareness of the current SNAFU (Situation Normal, All Frocked Up). It is the male role, in particular, that is held up to the mirror as Pentagon generals grudgingly acknowledge the contributions of gay men in the military; Robert Bly scores a huge best-seller with *Iron John*, in which men are encouraged to beat the bush and find their origins in Mother Nature; and authors such as Warren Farrell, PhD, question the myth of male power.

Remember the headlines that shrieked the scandal of 'nannygate' because the women whom President Clinton had nominated for the position of Attorney-General had employed illegal housekeepers? More than a hundred years after suffragettes fought for women's rights and planted the seeds of the feminist movement, women were still plagued with babysitter problems. Yet I was housemother to a unique sir-ority, many of whom envied the 1950s housewife and yearned to be in her place. At Miss Vera's Finishing School For Boys Who Want To Be Girls, we do our best to iron out the nation's domestic problems.

Students of the Academy, most of whom identify as heterosexual, are not Broadway babies or drag queens, though that is the level of expertise to which many aspire. The great drag performer, Divine, is one of the Academy's patron saints. Drag queens, who are usually gay, work it every day. They constantly perfect their performance personae. Students of the Academy do not. They are often married and well established in their occupations. But as cross-dressers, they have been touched with a heavy dose of the same magic that inspires the drag queen and made the shamans dance, the power of the combined masculine and feminine energies alive within each of us.

My book is an attempt to bring Miss Vera's Finishing School directly to the reader, with the same care and style we devote to each lucky neophyte who finds his way to our door. In essence, it is our Academy textbook. Perhaps you are a man who identifies as our students do. Like thousands of other men, you may have been dressed in girl's clothes when you were a child and those early experiences have inspired the creation of your female persona – or, as we call that amalgam of feelings and needs, your femmeself. You want to know more about her. Take a look at her. Help her to be the best she or he can be. The Academy can show you how. Maybe you are the wife or partner of a male cross-dresser who would like to be more informed for the purpose of enhancing your emotional and your sex life. The Academy will help you to do that, too.

I want to help more women – GGs or genetic girls as we call ourselves at the Academy – to understand and appreciate male cross-dressers. I and the other deans find ourselves the subjects of schoolgirl crushes from a whole group of very eligible bachelorettes and we want to share the wealth.

Perhaps you are a man who is simply curious to see how the other half lives. Even a man who has never had the desire to see himself in a skirt can benefit from the lessons of our Academy. In the process he will come to understand not only the ways in which men differ from women but the ways in which we are similar.

A former boyfriend who did not cross-dress once said to me, 'I wish I could be a woman for a while. If I were, I'd be able to wrap men around my little finger.' I have heard other men make similar claims. Usually they are convinced that given the right equipment, they could be *femmes fatales*. Here, we welcome all who want the chance to prove it.

Cross-dressing is an act that offers new options. Academy students learn to accommodate their shoes and take a rest from the rat-race. They discover how lipstick can colour their lives. Do not forget that while it is female clothing that is adopted, in many ways the clothing is merely a prop. The Academy dares the student to allow his male ego to be miss-taken and miss-guided.

It has been suggested that men like to cross-dress because it helps them to relieve stress. This far-too-simple explanation supports the myth of the dominant male and grossly underestimates female potency. Think about which values the female or Mother has supported compared to that of the male or Father. Traditionally Father represents strict adherence to rules of performance; Mother represents unconditional love. On the other hand, men know how to work; women know how to play. And Miss Vera knows how to play very well. Having grown up in the era of 'Father Knows Best' I know that 'Girls Just Want to Have Fun'. One way to define the Academy is to say that our business is education and recreation. We teach people to have fun.

What you will find here is a step-by-step guide to a male-to-female transformation. Ours is the holistic approach. We emphasise the physical changes, but do not dismiss the underlying feelings; we pay attention to nylons and crinolines, but do not overlook the Freudian slips. Students spend several hours at a time with us, or several days. Courses include make-up application, herstory, girl talk, flirting fundamentals, ballet 1 and tutu, sex education, etiquette, home economics, field trips (our girls go everywhere!)... Most of these are excellent subjects for any man to know, no matter what his fashion statement.

I am very proud of our students. They offer me and the deans – each one an expert in her field – the uplifting support of a tightly laced corset. They are our mainstays. Miss Vera's Finishing School is not all brick and concrete, not even all lipstick and lace, but a living, breathing reality that rests in the hearts and high-heeled souls of its students and teachers.

Students of the Academy, when not dressed in female clothes, lead very traditional lives. Many are family men with very mainstream jobs. They come from all walks of life: professionals and proletarians, young and old, married and single. They come in all body types, and bring to the Academy different-sized endowments.

The femmeself, as a creature of the imagination, is born to be uninhibited emotionally and sexually. How far the invisible woman goes when she becomes a material girl depends on him. Some of our students entertain the idea that they might live full-time as a female, but for the majority this is a fantasy. By giving our student the opportunity to make his fantasy a reality, we help him to understand the difference.

Our goal at the Academy is to bring out the female persona for the purpose of learning from her. Listen to her voice. What does she have to say? What does she like to do? How does she feel? What does she need, and where will she shop for it? We put the clothes in the closet and let the girl out.

For a long time, I have lived my life as the student, taking in information. Now that I am the teacher, I find that I still learn from my students. One of the things they have taught me is an appreciation of the power and passion of the female. Miss Vera's Finishing School has also helped to balance my energies. Assuming my role of Dean of Students has given me more creative outlets, more assurance, more financial security than I have ever known. Putting men in dresses has enabled me to wear the pants in my own life.

What has it done for the men? Often, even after the orientation interview, a student arrives for his first class and make-over with his face in a tight grimace of nerves. How gratifying it is to see that same student emerge with a grin that spreads from earring to earring. He has taken a brave step. Most of our students have never shared this side of themselves with anyone. It is a privilege for us to be with him at that moment when he is literally facing his greatest desire and his greatest fear in the mirror and to help him see that she is beautiful.

For years the man who enjoyed 'feminine pursuits' has been labelled a 'sissy'. At the Academy, we believe in sissy power. Our students' determination to free themselves and their feelings helps to liberate us all. In his quest to expand the idea of what it is to be masculine by embracing, celebrating and surrendering to the feminine influence, each student helps to expand the idea of who we are as humans. As we step boldly toward the new millennium, I am glad to know that many more of us will be doing it in high heels.

Our girls sometimes have difficulty answering these questions, but some answers they know by heart. They may not know one perfume from another, but our ladies-in-waiting all know what kind of car they drive. Most of the time it's a cherry-red Mustang convertible.

Homework Assignment #1: CREATE A HERSTORY

Dear Lady-in-Waiting, By answering the questions in the homework assignment 'Create A Herstory' you are encouraged to see your femmeself not simply as your own Barbie, but as a human with talents, characteristics and potential.

The following questions will help you discover the personality of your femmeself. Use details that describe not only who you are, but who you would like to be. In other words, your responses can be based on fact or fantasy. Let your femmeself choose the answers. Your responses can be used in planning your classes. Have fun!

- What is your age?
- How do you support yourself?
- How do you spend most of your time? Hobbies? Work?
- What are your favourite colours?
- Which fashion designers are your favourite? (If you cannot think of designers, try looking at *Harpers* and *Vogue*.)
- Which is your favourite perfume? (Sample them in department stores.)
- Do you have any galpals? What are they like?
- Do you date? Men? Women?
- Are you a virgin?
- If not, what is your sexual experience?
- Is there someone special in your life?
- What kinds of music do you prefer?
- What sort of entertainment do you like?
- Do you read? What?
- Which is your favourite season and why?
- If you could live anywhere in the world, where would you choose?
- If you could live during any period in history, which would it be?Do you participate in sports? Which ones?
- What is your favourite style of home decoration? (Some examples: Early American, 1950s retro, French Provincial, Louis XIV, Japanese modern etc.)
- Do you live alone?
- Do you own a car? If so, what kind?
- What do you like to eat?
- Do you cook? Are there other skills often associated with

females that you want to nourish in your femmeself? (Examples: sewing, housekeeping, childcare, hostessing, dancing, sexiness, making art, feminist activism, gardening...)

•Which female movie stars most appeal to you and why?Who are your favourite famous male hunks?

•Who are your female role models? Which other well-known or known only to you women, living or dead, do you admire, and why?

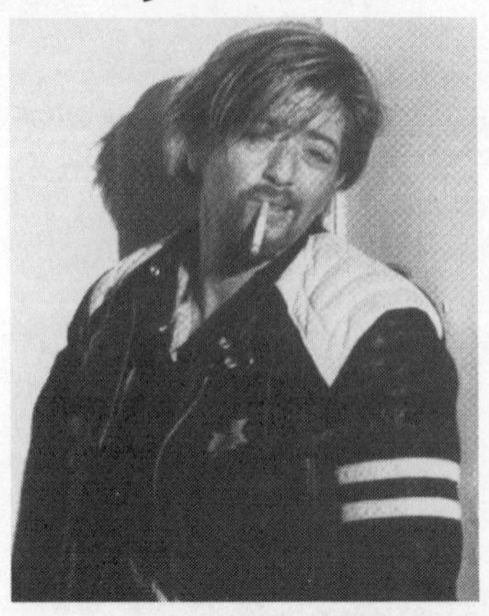

SHELLY MARS

Exploring your inner male

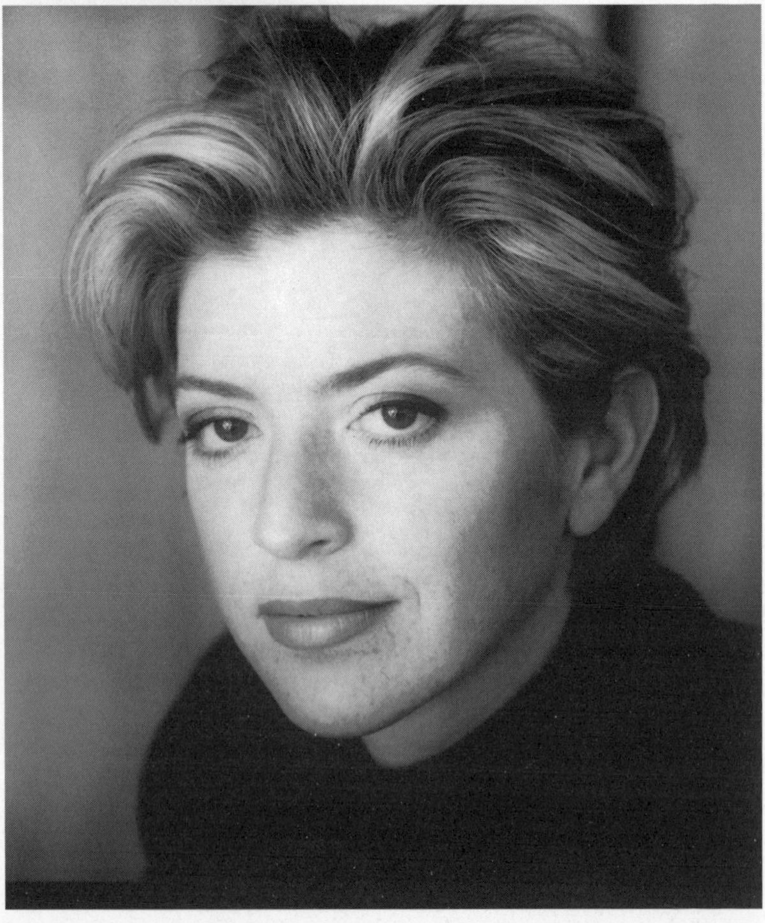

Shelly Mars is an actress and performance artist and has been described as the 'Lucille Ball of the 1990s' with a 'Robin Williams energy anchored by strong sexuality'. She is a powerful comic performer who aims to push herself and her audience beyond their limits. Known for her creation of male characters, particularly 'Martin', a stereotypical sexist heterosexual male. She runs drag king workshops and teaches women how to access their 'inner male'.

Shelly writes and stages her own material, produces and hosts a monthly comedy club talent showcase, 'Life on Mars', and works professionally as an actress and voiceover artist. She has a BFA in theatre from Cal Arts, and also studied at the American Conservatory Theatre. She currently teaches Performance Art for the Learning Annex in New York and tours nationally throughout the US with her one-woman shows.

I grew up as a tomboy, sometimes wanting to be a boy and spending a lot of time being around many guys, whom I both liked and hated. I always found some sort of conflict with men, it was almost torture, but I also really related to them too.

I think my trouble with men pushed me into becoming a performance artist. My public performance work, as a drag king creating male characters, came out of these feelings. I thought I wanted to be a movie or stage actress, but I realised that it would be more therapeutic to express myself on a more personal level. I obviously had a need to do it and I think people are attracted to the personal message of one-person shows.

Many women feel uncomfortable dealing with their masculine energy. One way you can embrace it is by creating a male persona. I created a male character called Martin as a way to deal with all the anger I had with men, probably not even knowing the level of my anger. When I took on this character I felt very powerful – I felt what it was like to be in a man's skin and expressed this. It was sexual and powerful and allowed me to play at being a male chauvinist pig. I realised that this was freedom and it became very therapeutic for me. I got to play with what I hated, and embrace it and own it.

I think that when you do something you fear, or have great disgust for, you learn how to embrace it and it becomes ingrained. Most of my characters are different colours on the palette of me; each different character is a different emotional me. Martin is the male chauvinist pig in Shelly. Over the years I learned that all of that was within me.

I think that all women can benefit from exploring their inner male. We are born with both male and female sides, and the world would be a better place if women knew their inner male; they would then know how to deal better with men. It is my theory that women can become any kind of man they want. I have many inner males – heterosexual, bisexual and gay, as well as sensitive men and outright pig males. As I get more sophisticated in working with male characters I have got to know the other males that live within me.

To me it's all about balance. If I'm wearing jeans and a sloppy T-shirt, feeling very boyish for days on end, then I need to wear a dress for a while to balance out the gender play inside of me. It is the same with my work and with my characters. If I play Martin or another male character a lot, it feels hideous – very imbalanced, and I want to do something very different to balance out the energy.

I am not always clear on my sexuality. It shifts all the time, so I explore it in my work. I am not confused. As I am bisexual I feel a need to sexually enjoy both sexes. When I am around many lesbians I want to be around men. When I am around men I want to be with women. I need balance in my life, I don't like to be around one type of person.

I love making love with women and I am just learning to enjoy it with men. It is not something I have loved for years, but now I am learning that through all the gender exploration I have been practising for years and the work I've done, something has been healed.

Creating these male characters has also been a way to investigate my own sexuality, to know what it is like to be with a woman, strap a dildo on and have a dick, and feel like a man in bed. It has also shown me what it feels like to take a dick, to play at being a boyfriend.

DIANE TORR

Any Woman can take on the role of a man

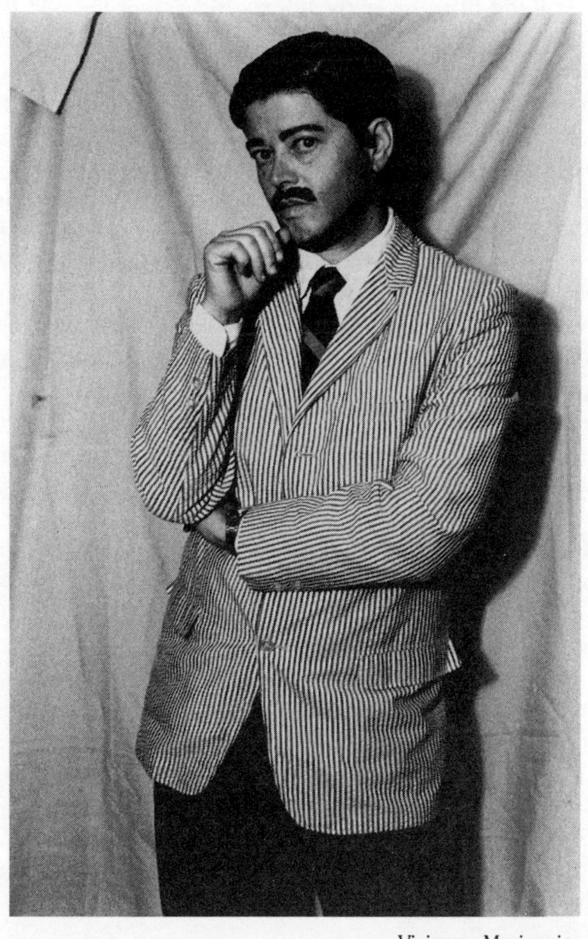

Vivienne Maricevic

Diane Torr is a performance artist and 'drag king ambassador' who has taught drag king workshops since 1989 throughout the US, England, Scotland, Germany, Switzerland, Austria, Holland, Scandinavia, and most recently in Istanbul, Turkey. In 2000, she will be giving workshops in Germany, England, Austria, New York and she will make a performance tour of Japan, were she will also be teaching workshops.

Contact Diane by writing to her at: dragkingdt@aol.comor at P.O. Box 481, New York, New York 10009

When I give a Drag King Workshop, it is a whole-day experience sometimes going into the early hours of the morning. At first the workshop was at Annie Sprinkle's Salon on Lexington Avenue and East 26th Street, New York. In a way the whole drag king scene began when Johnny Armstrong, who did the make-up, and I began teaching the workshop there in 1989. Johnny also organised drag king contests at local venues like the Pyramid Club and we were invited to appear on talk-shows, such as the Donahue show in 1991.

It was exciting to see how the phrase 'drag king' gradually became included in the vernacular and the concept of female-to-male cross-dressing becoming part of everyday life. People stopped saying, 'I've heard of drag queens, but what's a drag king?' and instead of thinking I led 'Dry cleaning workshops', people actually heard, and comprehended the phrase 'drag king workshops'.

Since the late 1980s, we have presented workshops in many different locales – Annie's Salon, art spaces, theatre rehearsal studios, private apartments, lofts. I've toured the workshop and presented it at places where I also happened to be performing. I have led hundreds of women through the experience of female-to-male cross-dressing, teaching the workshop in the US, Canada and Europe.

The response varied from city to city, from country to country. For some it was a continuation of their own exploration, and for others, it was a once-only experience. The workshop has pioneered a way for women to take on a male identity and live as men for a day, and to take the exploration further in their daily lives, if they so wish.

I have worked with women of every sexual persuasion – straight, gay, bisexual, celibate, asexual and practically every ethnicity and age group. I've had a girl of eleven attend the workshop, and a woman of sixty-nine, and all the ages in between. I would say the workshop is of universal interest.

I plan next to bring the workshop to Istanbul to work with Muslim women and then to Ireland and Japan to work with women in rural areas there.

For the most part, the participants of the drag king workshop are women who want to try out another gender. Women have taken the workshop who wanted to use the disguise to their advantage, as in buying a car, for example, or to gain entry to places and situations that would be difficult to access as women. The idea of creating a male alter ego is a useful strategy, for instance, for women who want to travel alone in countries where women of any age are sexual targets.

Some women are performers and actresses, and want to expand their repertoire. There were many workshop participants who took the workshop as a kind of assertiveness training. They also wanted to learn the kind of behaviour that men adopt in order to assume a sense of privilege and entitlement. Others simply wanted to 'own their space'. Many took the workshop for sexual frisson. They arranged to meet their boyfriend or girlfriend at the conclusion of the workshop for a night of sexual role-switching and fun.

The thing to realise is that any woman can take on the role of a man. Gender is not immutable, which means that no matter how femme you think you are, there is the opportunity to construct the masculine, if that's what you want to do. And it can be a lot of fun. In the course of constructing a masculine identity, women learn other possibilities of being, and this can only enhance your sex life.

Behaviour that you felt you could never do as 'Cathy' is immediately accessible as 'Bill'. Places you'd never consider going, like a beach at four in the morning on a hot summer's night, suddenly become available to you. This allows for a whole new adventure in flirting and playing around. Cruising, for instance, takes on a different meaning and flavour when you assume a male identity.

Every woman has imagined herself as a man. How can she not? In a world where we have constantly been seen as 'other', we have been taught to be a spectacle for the male gaze. What does 'he' want to see? How can I construct myself to be appealing or desirable? Or, in rebelling against that self-consciousness, we fought hard to be our own persons. In defining ourselves, we have adopted so-called 'masculine' behaviour such as having a sense of our own space, or feeling the right to speak out and demand to be heard, or speaking as if we mean what we say, not constantly apologising or smiling to appease.

There are also women who mix and match behaviour so that in the work situation, for instance, she might perform a set of acceptable gestures, responses, routines, and in her leisure time, she becomes someone else. Women have learned, for the purposes of survival, to be observant. We learn what every nuance of male gesture signifies. If you grew up with elder brothers as I did, you had to watch out that they wouldn't gang up against you. This meant that I developed serious observation skills. All this observation and 'watching out' has meant that women have learned – almost through osmosis – male gestures, mannerisms, behaviours. It is surprising how quickly women assume the masculine; it is almost as if this material is there already, just waiting to be exposed.

EXERCISE: CREATING YOUR OWN DRAG KING WORKSHOP

The creation of a male identity, like many things, depends very much on your commitment to the investigation. You need a space with plenty of room so you can strut about. Mirrors, so you can be constantly reminded of who you have become. Manly music like heavy metal or 'Macho Man' if you want to take the piss. Beers, snacks and most important, attitude.

When thinking about the male identity you wish to construct, be very attentive to the type of clothes that man would wear. If you don't think it through, you will feel awkward and uncertain in your male persona. Your outward appearance will convey much of what you think of yourself as a man.

Here is a list of potential male personae you may want to consider: corporate executive, dandy, mechanic, gay boy, computer nerd, advertising executive, rock musician, macho playboy, waiter, biker, hippy, punk, art boy, academic, labourer, salesman. Each of these male characters has particular orientations that can be explored in sexual play with a partner.

Facial hair is the big signifier in creating a male identity. Even if your tits are showing and you're wearing a dress, if you're also packing a moustache, chances are if you're out and about, people will think you are a male transsexual. If that's your male identity, go right ahead.

However, other men wear suits, leather or sportswear and with a moustache or whiskers or goatee and sideburns, you have a better opportunity to blend in. You can get facial hair from a theatre make-up or novelty store.

If you look closely at men's facial hair (and it is possible to stare at men for long periods of time without them noticing) you will see that often it is compiled of different shades. So, mix the hair shades for a more authentic look. Prepare the facial hair by cutting it into small bits. Use spirit gum to create the shape of the moustache, sideburns or goatee on your face and then apply the small bits of hair. It takes practice to get this looking good. To create symmetrical sideburns, do them one at a time. Eyebrows can be thickened with mascara, but if you pluck, you may need to add facial hair to fill in the gaps. It is important to add the five o'clock shadow after the facial hair because traces of spirit gum are sometimes left on the skin and you need to clean that up before you do the shadow, otherwise it gets patchy. You can use something that professionals use – a blush brush and dark brown or black eye-shadow (make sure it's matt and doesn't contain sparkly bits).

Don't forget the neck. If you examine men's necks, you'll see that the shadow is stronger along the edge of the lower jawbone. You can also emphasise with dark shadow, bags that you may already have under your eyes. Men don't have the worries women are supposed to have about accumulating signs of age and haggardness. It may even enhance your male appearance and give you that rugged look!If you have long hair, either comb it back and hold it with a rubber band at the nape of the neck – let the hair hang limply down the back. If you are going to let your hair hang loose, try parting your hair in the middle rather than at the side. If you think your hair still doesn't look right, try adding some hair gel. Experiment with combing your hair in a different style, play around with your look. Whatever length or type of hair you have, you can be sure there is a male with the same.

For breast binding wind a 10-12cm-wide elastic bandage around your torso, starting at the base of the breasts and covering the nipples first. It's useful to have someone help you as you need to distribute the bandage evenly, without creasing, as once you move around any creases can bunch up, and your breasts may pop out! The binding should be secure but not so tight that you have difficulty breathing. If you have large breasts, you may need two elastic bandages, in which case, they should overlap slightly, so there isn't a gap between them.

If, after binding, you feel like your breasts still register too much of a bulge, put on a shirt and you'll see you've suddenly acquired pronounced pectoral muscles!There are many ways to construct a fake penis. Some people use condoms stuffed with cotton wool, others have used rolled-up socks, others a banana or a dildo. You may wish to titillate your partner by unzipping your fly to reveal your 'manhood' and playing with this toy together. Or you may wish to have just the suggestion of a bulge, which can also be arousing to look at and to stroke.

Shoes – don't try to get away with women's sports shoes – they aren't unisex. Men's shoes are wider and more roomy than women's. When you put on men's shoes, you feel as if you are fully standing on the earth and owning the space under your feet. This strong physical contact with the ground has a consequent psychological effect. Experience it.

I've based my behaviour observations on a stereotyped white, middle-class American male. This is because, unfortunately, stereotypes represent the norm, or what can be identified as 'typically male'. Your character may not be like this description, but you can extrapolate from this information what might be useful to you.

It is important to stop smiling. Right now. As women we smile frequently to make ourselves appear unthreatening and so that people can feel comfortable in our company. Men generally don't smile as much as women – they smile when there is a reason to smile.

Practise opaqueness so that you are impervious to even the most penetrating stare. If you need help in understanding this, watch any grey-haired man in a suit – a sense of power and purpose is conveyed in his dress, body language, gesture and facial expression. When you walk into a room as a man in a suit, people take notice of you. You are accorded significance without even opening your mouth or doing anything.

You are expected to be arrogant and forceful because, as a man in a man's world, you are right! Even if you're not, never admit it, and don't apologise. Expect to be treated with respect and privilege, and never show signs of uncertainty or discomfort, because this could be construed as not being in charge, and it is most important that you maintain authority at all times.

When you walk, jut your feet out to the side. The action comes from the shoulders. Hips are frozen and are led by the swing in the shoulders from side to side. As you walk, take up a lot of space as you are letting your weight fall first to one side and then the other. Not only do you take up space as you walk, but also think of an additional perimeter of about one metre around your body, as your territory. Anyone who steps into your boundary is looking for trouble. As you walk and do most actions, your hands are held in a semi-clenched position. Sometimes they hang in your pockets. Then the arms hang down too, and are bent at the elbow.

Sit with your legs wide apart and your feet planted firmly on the floor. If your legs protrude into another person's seat space (as on a subway train, for example) that's not your problem. If you are not reading a newspaper, use your folded hands to rest in front of your cock. If you cross your legs, you make a figure 4 shape with the ankle resting on the knee of one bent leg. When you sit down, adjust your pants by pulling up the creases at the knees, just before you take your seat. Then sink down deep with your arse touching the back of the chair. Never sit on the edge of the seat – that's what women do. When you get up from the chair, take your time. Don't spring up. Lean forward, straighten up and take a step.

In developing a male persona, you will need to discover certain abilities that you never developed as a woman. Being able to stare 'through' someone is a good example. As a woman, when a man stares at you, you automatically look down and avert your gaze because you don't want to enter into a confrontation with that person, unless you are attracted to him or her, and then you might return the gaze. As a man, learn to look at people as if your gaze is initiated from deep inside your head, and give off a sense of self-reserve.

When you talk, try to keep your voice low in tone, yet use the voice with volume. Most importantly, don't raise your voice at the end of a sentence as if asking a question. Be direct, and speak in categorical statements, as if you have the definitive answer. If your talk is accompanied by appropriate significant gestures, you will be seen to be male.

Gestures are specific and direct and used to emphasise rather than embellish. Gestures might include pointing with the forefinger or be seen to slice the air with two hands just about mid-chest level – as in the phrase 'I've had it with this job'. One gesture of poignancy and determination is to punch the palm of one hand with the fist of the other. This is a gesture you can use only once during a conversation; if you use it more often, it loses power and authority.

Men very rarely touch their bodies, unless it's to adjust their balls or to hit the sides of the thighs as an expression of finality. Some gestures to consider:

• standing with your feet together, lift up your heels and let them drop down with a click
• jangle loose change in your pocket
• pretend to listen to someone and then shrug your shoulders in a gesture of disinterest
• fold the arms and recede the head and chest while somebody is grappling to express themselves
• unbutton your jacket and put one thumb in the waist of your pants, and use the other hand to point with your finger.

As you can see, performing as a man can be quite enjoyable and may push you to delve into your inner resources. Gender is an act. Whereas femininity is perceived always as drag, no matter who is wearing it, which is why it is so easy to caricature, maleness is the presumed universal. This being the case, you can see how maleness seems less artificial. This is to women's advantage as it will be easier to pass in the male guise when we are out having a good time at the places we would perhaps never go to as women, such as strip bars or go-go clubs.

Maleness is assumed unless proven otherwise. Consequently, even if you feel you don't pass, the fact that you've entered into this transgressive act and are performing as a male is sufficient. You have the possibility to create the person of your dreams – someone who will act on your wildest sexual fantasies – and who may reveal desires that you never knew you had. In performing the masculine, you give yourself the opportunity to expand, to go beyond the allotted 'female' roles that have been apportioned to us.

I started becoming interested in male roles when, as a young girl, I became aware of the fact that my brothers were treated differently from me. Fortunately, one of my brothers (who later turned out to be gay) and I formed a conspiracy to subvert our parents' expectations of us. He would do the dusting and I would dig in the garden. He would push my dolls and pram around the block and I would make a building with his Lego.

Later, when I became involved with the feminist movement in London in 1968 I did further research and reading on ideas of gender difference. By studying dance and theatre, I became involved in examining ideas of androgyny through movement. The first performance was in 1982 in New York. My character was a Jean-Paul Belmondo type and my friend played a pregnant Vietnamese woman, who had recurred in his dreams. I also created a boy/woman strip act that I performed at various clubs in New York between 1978 and 1983. Many of the theatre performances I've presented in the past fifteen years have involved the development of different male characters. I have six male identities I've been messing about with over the years.

I've also constructed spur-of-the-moment characters for club gigs. This public appearance of gender exploration has affected my personal exploration of gender and sexuality? I am much more open to play with roles. In sexual play, it can be liberating to put on costumes and become someone else. I am very skilled at that. My girlfriend loves it! We both dress in drag and go out as two gay men, or I'll be a woman one time and she the guy, or vice versa. It definitely adds to our sex life.

norrie mAy -welby

Like a bridge over the sex divide

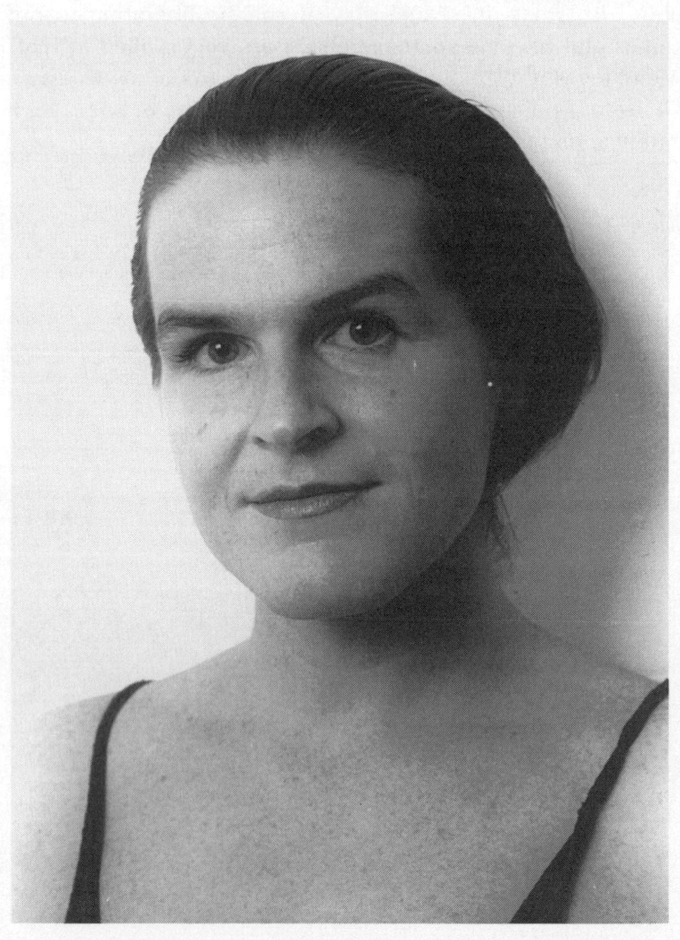

norrie mAy-welby was born with more capitals and a slightly different shape to hir name, which was no less true of hir body. (Since norrie is of no single fixed gender, I have used androgynous pronouns, that is, 'hir' for his or her, 'zie' for she or he and 'hirs' for hers or his.) Zie came to Perth, Western Australia with hir family as a ten-pound tourist, in a scheme designed to prop up the monocultural values of White Australia. Since then, zie has since been working almost non-stop to build a culture that values diversity, freedom of expression and sex positivity (or, in other words, to undermine and destroy the dominant culture she was imported to promote).

norrie has been a published writer since high school, working hir own bent on sexuality into Perth's university and gay press. Zie moved to Sydney in 1988, joined the management committee of the Australian Transsexual Association (a welfare organisation) and became co-ordinator of the more politically oriented Transgender Liberation Coalition. Zie co-presented a radical workshop on gender, transgender and feminism at the 1991 Queer Collaborations conference, and with hir co-presenter, Aidy Griffin, wrote the ground-breaking 'Gender Agenda' columns in the Sydney Star Observer.

norrie has written, performed and taught in gender, sexuality and transgender in various forums and media, including the 3rd International Congress on Sex and Gender (Oxford University, 1998), the New South Wales high school curriculum book Girl Talk (1998) and the television documentaries On Becoming *and* Sexing the Label. *Zie is currently working with the Sex Workers Outreach Project.*

I thank the Goddess I was labelled a male at birth, or else I may never have been able to find any sympathy for men. It would seem to me, from my body's topography and eruptions, that I even had a normal amount of testosterone when I was a teenager.

However, this failed to dispose me toward violence, rape or any other uncontrollable passions. Nor did I have any appreciation for the notion that male and female humans were different species, and that exploitation and manipulation of one by the other was acceptable practice.

This idealistic idyll was shaken up when I found my self-expression disapproved and penalised by an adult workplace that imposed gender conformity. My self-expression was classified as 'female' and prohibited for one of apparently male physiognomy. To cut a long story (among other things) short, I changed my physiognomy, and asserted a female social identity. This did not seem to me to be a change of gender, for I had never had a sense of myself as male, merely a 'natural' affirmation of my inherent femaleness. Of course, this affirmation was only made necessary because of a social insistence on either male or female gender identification.

When I was about ten, I had crushes on a couple of girls, but I was thoroughly disenchanted by the gender roles that were expected in opposite sex relations. I wanted to be treated as an equal, not a transparent klutz with a fixed agenda to be manipulated and exploited. I also had a crush on a boy at about this age, and idly wondered if this meant I was homosexual.

I had another long-lasting crush on a boy during my mid-teens, and consequently identified as gay. My initial sexual interactions were less definitive however, since some of my partners were male, some female, and my behaviour ranged from normal heterosexual male to passive homosexual, to throw around some clinical labels.

I rigidly policed my behaviour as a pre-op transsexual to make sure I would qualify for genital realignment surgery. I sought this partly because I believed the popular notion that one's public gender should be properly reflected in the gender of one's privates. I bought the idea that has oppressed women since the advent of advertising, that we should all aspire to have the one ideal type of female body. I even came to believe that there were 'proper' ways for women to behave, tolerated no departure from this in myself, and took pride in my conformity to ideas of femininity.

I then found I was the sort of woman who was treated very badly by straight men, and became open to the idea of changing what sort of woman I was. I explored personal development books and courses, freed myself from the bounds of pre-existing self-notions, and allowed myself to express all that was in me as a whole human, without regard to gender limitations. Of course, being a whole woman is not essentially different from simply being a whole person.

When I identified myself as female and lived as transsexual, almost all my partners were male, although their own identifications ranged from straight to bisexual to gay (much as they had when I was a garden-variety gay boy). A few lesbians tried to seduce me too. As I wasn't bound by a fear of homosexuality (having been happily a gay male), many of these seductions were consummated.

Now that I have grown beyond standard gender limitations, I am not only fluid in my social gender, but also play with gender in intimate interactions. I am confident enough in my femininity to wear a strap-on without feeling that this compromises my womanhood. I have rejected any shame about being transgender, and being visible about this spares me from involvement with sexually insecure, sexist and homophobic men. I've also experienced the sexual attraction inherent in gender ambiguity, and consummated relations with a few transgender people of various gender types.

I have since found myself at the forefront of gender and transgender politics, negotiating practical solutions for gender-gifted people in gender-restricted situations, while working toward the ideal where no-one is persecuted or treated as inferior because of their gender status. As long as there are men and women who think the other sex is an alien race, as long as intersexed children (hermaphrodite) are denied the gender they were born with, as long as people are persecuted for the sake of 'gender norms', I will continue to work for the destruction of gender tyranny.

As a transgendered person, some people (and some laws) see me as male, some as female, some as 'not male', some as 'not female'. Sometimes I may experience myself as masculine, sometimes as feminine. Whether I am essentially a male or female person is like asking the planet whether it is essentially a day person or a night person.

Finding standard gender terms ill-fitting, I coined my own term to reflect my own gender position. This term is 'spansexual': 'sex' comes from the Latin seco, to divide, and I span the division. Like a bridge, I am located in both places at once, and I've travelled from one side to the other. Like a bridge over the sex divide, I overlook the space between the sexes, and I can see each side from both sides.

The sexes are not poles apart. They may be on different sides of the equator, but the equator is just an 'imaginary' line. 'Spansexual' applies, then, not just to bridging the divisions of sex, but to bridging any and all harmful divisions.

Society has made many divisions within and between us. Divisions of race, sex, age, class, colour, sexuality and divisions between ourselves and our environment. I believe that we can honour our unique differences without being separate from each other, that we can express any particular aspect of ourselves without disowning other aspects, and that we can live as part of our environment, not 'apart' from it. I believe that health and lasting happiness come from wholeness, not separateness.

I have been a sex worker and this has put me in many situations that I may never have explored on my own initiative. While some of these activities have not been things that held any appeal for me outside of my profession, some have become part of my personal sexual practice. It was also as a sex worker that I began intuitively practising techniques such as channelling sexual energy for healing in a Reiki-like manner, that I later learned were part of New Age Tantric practices. Tantra now plays part of both my sex work and my personal life.

Having had sex with such a wide range of people has led to an experience-based understanding of the mindboggling diversity of human sexuality. Having encouraged so many people to be accepting of and to explore their individual inclinations, it would have been hypocritical if I had not encouraged myself to do the same. I don't blink if I find myself entertaining a sexual attraction or fantasy that I can't easily understand or see precedents for.

As an amateur, I was often treated as an unpaid sex worker. Now that I was getting paid for 'Wham bam thank you ma'am', I had higher expectations of recreational intimacy. I became much more assertive about getting my own needs met.

Before I began any conscious personal development work, I saw myself as an isolated being who was dependent on others' approval. I was always endeavouring to meet their expectations, and trying to conform to their idea of 'normality'. Since then, I have been more conscientious about being true to myself, whether or not this gains outside validation.

In exploring who I was and could be as a woman, I have also explored and developed aspects that I had formerly labelled 'masculine' and therefore inappropriate. I have reclaimed and rejoiced in Artemis within me. It does seem that my current *yin–yang* flux is mostly yin, that is, female, and has been this way for most, if not all, of this lifetime. I still maintain, however, a commonality with everyone on the sex – gender continuum. There is no fundamental difference between other women and me, or between me and an effeminate queen, or between the queen and a bisexual man, or between a bisexual man and a straight man.

I have chosen to reject sex-negative values, and been critical of 'moral' and 'religious' restrictions on physical pleasure and sexuality. It seems to me that these restrictions are designed to keep us from our personal power and pleasure, to make us dependent on external authority. I experience my sensuality and sexuality as divine gifts that can unite me with myself, with other people, and with the physical and spiritual world I am part of.

The more connected I allow myself to be with the seen and unseen energies within and around me, the more these energies flow to, through, around and within me. The more I trust that the universe I am part of will look after its own, the less my ego stresses out trying to manage the universe. The less division I allow between myself and other people, whether of gender, race, class or whatever, the more I experience my connection to all of humanity and to all of the human that I am.

EXERCISE: DOING GENDER PLAY

As different as male and female bodies seem to be, the similarities are even more astounding. Each sexual feature seems to have a counterpart in the other sex. Yet men quite often have their nipples and G-spot ignored, while women may find their external genitals overlooked. Making love to a man without touching his G-spot is as rude as making love to a woman without touching her clitoris.

Where's his G-spot, you may wonder. Well, I'm talking about the 'masculinis uterus' (male womb), located on the prostate gland. This can be stimulated by a finger or dildo in his anus, but penetration is not essential.

The male G-spot is accessible on the perineum, that little seam between the scrotum and anus. Follow the penis down past its base to its root, and you'll find that just below the scrotum, the root of the penis curves back in to the body. There's a soft spot between this erectile tissue and the anus. Pressing here will generate the same sort of sensations as a woman would get from her G-spot being fingered. (It may be more pleasant to do this with very short fingernails.)You may find it fun to play with gender roles, regardless of the sex or social gender identity of your partner. Swapping roles can be a way of increasing intimacy, as you actually experience what your partner usually experiences, and vice-versa. Not every man will be comfortable with being told 'Yes, baby, suck my beautiful dick' when he's got the tip of your clit in his mouth, but turnabout is fair play, I say. Role-play is not limited to straight role reversal. Lesbians may have fun impersonating a heterosexual couple, or playing the roles of gay males, and a heterosexual couple may imagine themselves as a lesbian pair. Imagine that 'clitoris' is just another name for 'penis', 'labia' for 'scrotum', and remember everyone's got a G-spot and nipples!

4

Women Scribes and Educators

In the past women writers frequently took a male *nom de plume*, to guarantee being published and read. The Brontë sisters, for example, published their first book of poems under the names Currer, Ellis and Acton Bell. For women to write about sexuality was especially taboo. Yet women have most often illuminated a changing sexual landscape and have seen female sexual experience as an erotic signpost of the social freedom of the times. This is seen in the work of such writers as Anaïs Nin, Colette, Sylvia Plath and Simone de Beauvoir.

Many writers, even novelists, are unintentional educators. By describing where society is, and where it has been, they open up the possibility of pointing to where society may be going. Books, magazines and newspapers travel and the ideas expressed in one part of the world can easily be taken up in another, making every sexuality writer a potential educator. Publications are passed between friends, reach a wide audience and help to spread information.

Previously primary information on sexuality came from the medical profession. Psychologists, therapists (New Age and traditional) and lifestyle writers are now just as likely to dispense valuable sexual advice as your local doctor.

Women writers also turned their gaze on the erotic imagination and in the 1970s new collections of racy short stories, full-length sex novels and feminist pornography appeared. For the first time erotica was written from a female point of view, with women and men described through the eyes of a woman. Desire, sexual destiny and fantasies were reshaped.

One of the most important aspects of second wave feminism was the rise of independent feminist publications and female-owned and controlled presses. These early women's presses printed the earliest sexual self-help manuals, women's health publications and collections of woman-orientated erotic stories. Lesbian magazines soon followed and the appearance of *On Our Backs*, a parody of popular feminist magazine *off our backs*, in 1984 in the US changed the public landscape of female desire forever. It was the inspiration for many magazines which followed, from the UK's *Quim* to *Australia's Wicked Women.*

Whole new areas of sexuality were opened up for discussion through these new women-owned and controlled publications and this flowed over into the new heterosexual women's magazines such as Australian Women's Forum and New Woman. Together they proved there was a market eager for a woman's perspective on sexual exploration and education.

For women who were socially isolated such publications had the effect of enhancing their view of the world. They had different images of women presented to them, the writing of the newest writers on emerging women's sexuality and access to the phone numbers and the new emerging women's sexuality businesses.

Although women's sex shops were opening, with products designed for a woman's body, it was the support offered by female sexuality writers that contributed to the change of consciousness that made the success of these businesses possible. Before a woman could walk into a women's sex shop and buy a vibrator, dildo or other sex toy, she had to have an expanded view of her sexuality that made her believe that this would be a positive thing to do.

Another new development since the 1970s is the number of female writers who have been workers in the sex industry, from strippers to dominatrixes, who have put their lives and their opinions of the industry on paper. These new female sex writers are claiming ground in the discussions about prostitution and other forms of sex work, because they are coming from the perspective of workers in this industry.

However, just as they have forged new ground women writers have also felt the sting of censorship and have found their work banned or taken out of print. It is not surprising then to see many women sexuality writers and educators also active in anti-censorship campaigns. In this chapter Carol Queen, Kimberly O'Sullivan and Ruth Ostrow show how the nature of their work has often forced them to become free speech activists and educators in the area of erotic freedom.

CARROL QUEEN

Being present in your sexuality and pleasure

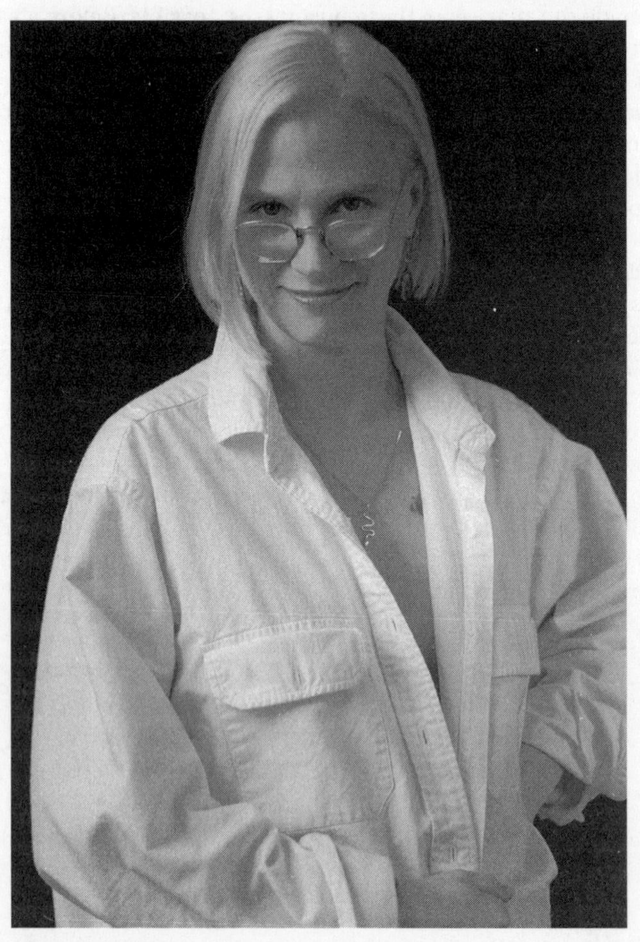

Layne Winklebleck

Carol Queen is a pleasure activist author, and sex educator who lives with her partner of ten years, Robert Morgan, in San Francisco. She is a cultural sexologist with a doctorate in education (EdD/sexology). Her erotic writing and cultural commentary have been widely anthologised.

Carol is especially known for writing about bisexuality, pornography, the sex industry, SM and other often-stigmatised erotic variations. She approaches these topics with the benefit of an academic background, but also knows them from the inside and openly discusses her personal experiences as well.

She is the author or co-editor of Exhibitionism for the Shy, Real Live Nude Girl, The Leather Daddy and the Femme, PoMoSexuals, Switch Hitters and Sex Spoken Here. *An acknowledged exhibitionist, Carol has also appeared in several explicit educational videos, including* Carol Queen's Great Vibrations: An Explicit Consumer Tour of Vibrators and Bend Over Boyfriend: A Couple's Guide to Male Anal Pleasure *(with her partner Robert). She is currently workshopping a solo performance called 'Peep Shop', based on her experiences in the sex industry.*

Carol is a worker-owner at Good Vibrations, where she directs continuing employee education and works with the marketing department. She also writes regularly for Libido *and* Spectator *magazines, and the East Bay Express, and teaches sex ed workshops.*

Her website is www.carolqueen.com.

I came out as bisexual at a pretty young age, fifteen. At that point I hadn't had sex with any women, but knew I wanted to. It was the early 1970s, when such experimentation and desire was looked upon as fairly acceptable – except in the gay/lesbian community. I felt close to that community politically, but when I arrived at its metaphoric doorstep I was pretty resoundingly rejected, or, rather, told I was 'going through a phase' and that I should 'pick one', men or women.

After hearing that enough times, I did – I chose women, partly because I thought I already knew what having sex with men was all about. (From this vantage point, now that I'm over forty, I can't believe I thought I'd experienced it all at the age of eighteen – but I was that uneducated, not even understanding that I had yet to fully grow into my own sexuality.)Besides, I understood intimacy (sexual and emotional) with women as very different from what I experienced with men, even though I hadn't been lovers with any women yet! The lesbian and feminist communities supported me, declaring that relating to women was very different from relating to men. Quite honestly, now that I've been bisexual for twenty-five years and have had both female and male lovers, I no longer think there are such substantial differences. But in any case, at that time, I had to follow where my desire and fascinations led me, and so I declared myself a lesbian and for the next decade had very little to do with men sexually.

At the end of that time I understood that relationships with women were not perfect or easy. I'd also come to understand that I would always have strong feelings for men. They were erotic feelings but also feelings of love – and what allowed me to understand this was the relationships I'd formed with gay men. Though I did not have sex with most of them, there were many men in my life whom I loved deeply. When the AIDS epidemic began to affect them, it pushed me into realising that by denying my feelings for men in order to fit into the lesbian community, I was doing myself a great disservice and not being whom I truly was, as surely as gays and lesbians stayed in the closet.

It wasn't that I didn't love and desire women. But I finally came to terms with my bisexuality in a deep rather than a superficial way. Since then I have always been out as bi (or, as I sometimes say, pansexual, since I think the term 'bisexual' implies that there are only two sexes/genders, and I believe there are many more than that). I have written extensively about bisexual issues, and most of my erotic writing, I believe, can be characterised as bisexual.

I live with a man, but we are not monogamous; we tend to want women in our lives who are in a relationship with both of us. We've had one such relationship that lasted eighteen months; she broke up with us to be in a monogamous relationship with another woman. It's often thought all bis have, or want, relationships like this – threesomes – and that's one reason bisexuals are sometimes misunderstood. How could a bi person be happy any other way, right? But most bisexuals are probably monogamous – it takes a good deal of skill and maturity for most people to be comfortably non-monogamous and I believe that the majority of bisexuals express their sexuality by having sex with women and men (and perhaps others!) over the course of many years – not all in a weekend!Having said this, it is also true that bisexuals have a reason to learn to be non-monogamous, if they choose, in a principled and mature way. If bisexuality is the capacity to desire women and men, perhaps you could say those of us who have women and men as lovers are experiencing our sexual potential in a deeper way. But there are so many variables in each person's sex and love life that I'm hesitant to make this claim.

Open relationships are not inherent to any sexual orientation; they are one way people of any orientation(s) can choose to structure relationships. And having what is sometimes called a 'responsible non-monogamous' orientation to relationships is not the same as indiscriminate promiscuity; promiscuity is a choice anyone might make, as are celibacy and monogamy. I should end by pointing out that promiscuity isn't always 'indiscriminate' either! Someone may want lots of sex with lots of partners, yet still be choosy about whom she or he will or won't have sex with, and what kind of sex she or he will have.

Anyone who has read my non-fiction or heard me speak about sex knows that I started out very shy – with lots of adventurous fantasies and desires, but very hesitant about finding ways to make them come true. I was nearly tongue-tied in bed, and many of my earliest sexual experiences were much the worse for it. But I was not happy this way. I knew sex would be better and I would be happier if I could get over my intense reticence. My first serious girlfriend helped me enormously; we were together for five years, long enough to get comfortable with talking, sharing and exploring fantasies, and getting a little exhibitionistic.

After coming to San Francisco I began to explore group sex, where I met my next two partners, both bisexual men. Coming out as bisexual, exploring SM, working in the sex industry, and doing all the other things I've done, including studying sexology, has situated me sexually in a far different place than the one I started out in – yet I can still recognise that girl whose wild fantasies have finally been lived out. Getting here was a long, step-by-step process, most of it, I'm happy to say, very pleasurable.

The most important thing I've learned on this journey: communicating is enormously important. If you can't do it, trouble will probably follow! But learning to communicate (about sex, about everything) is step-by-step, too, and it helps very much if you and your partner really want to be compatible and happy sexually and – is quite important – don't have too many preconceived ideas about what that means. I refer here especially to rigid, gender-based ideas of what is appropriate for men or women. In real life, our skills and interests may be shaped by gender roles, but often we cross that imaginary line, and it's okay to do so – it's much healthier than being restricted because 'women aren't interested in that' or 'men don't act that way'.

It is also not useful to compare yourself to others. It's hard not to – for one thing, that's what the whole emphasis on being sexually 'normal' is all about, which only engenders judgement and bias and even self-hatred. This sort of comparison is, I think, a root of women's and men's physical self-esteem problems. We often don't feel adequate and attractive because we compare ourselves with people in magazines, in advertisements, in movies. A hard lesson to learn is that often our partner wants us just the way we are, but we can get so hung up on not looking the way we think we should that it gets in the way of our sexual feelings and responses. Being present in your sexuality and pleasure is absolutely more attractive and erotically compelling than having a perfect body.

These sorts of role-based assumptions and failures to communicate help power the sex industry, in which partnered men pay others to give them what they think (sometimes correctly, other times not) their wives won't. The sex industry is used by single men too, but I know that a good percentage (almost certainly the majority) of my customers have wives or partners. If we can get over the sexual and gender double standards so that people could relate sexually on an equal basis, much of the sex industry would lose its relevance – or change to something not only men but women and partners could and would access.

I honour the sex industry – among other things, it gets (some) people's needs met and facilitates exploration, and the women and men who work in it are often courageous and extraordinary people. But I do not honour the fact that it is set up principally for men's entertainment.

I urge women to ask themselves, if I had the money, knew where to call a woman or a man to pleasure or entertain me, and knew it was safe to do so, what would I do? If you can't answer that, why not? A final thing I have learned: if you can't give yourself pleasure, if your sexuality is not centred in yourself, it's hopeless (and rather dangerous) to expect someone else to come along and awaken you like Prince Charming does Sleeping Beauty. Sometimes partners may awaken us, but they do not infuse us with sexuality. It is in each of us all along.

Fantasy and self-pleasure can get you in touch with who you are, regardless of who your partner is, who you are with him or her, or whether you have a partner at all. I think we not only have the option of exploring ourselves in this way, but we have a responsibility to do so, because we're then better able to communicate what we want and to take care of ourselves. Besides, it's so lonely and hopeless to think pleasure is only in our lives when someone else brings it to us. Pleasure can be with us every day.

TIPS ON EXHIBITIONISM

Here's what I'd recommend for someone who wants to get more comfortably exhibitionistic.

• First, show off for yourself. Pick a comfortable room where you have privacy, a mirror and enough room to move around. Turn the lights low or light candles if you like, but make sure you can still see. Put on sexy music that you like to dance to, and begin to move. Concentrate on how your body feels - even if you wouldn't feel comfortable in public with pelvis thrusts and lots of hip-swaying, do it here.

• Watch yourself in the mirror from time to time. Look for evidence of your own pleasure in the movement. Get into it, and appreciate how you look when you're in your body and happy to be there. Now, begin to take off your clothes. Make it slow, which looks sexier than flinging them off. The slower, the better. Tease and take all the time in the world. Reveal, then cover, now do it again. Keep moving to the music although there's no need to full-on dance while stripping; that can get rather complicated. Just keep some sway, some movement to it.

• Watch yourself at least sometimes, and not too judgementally, either. Be playful. For now, you are the only voyeur.

• Now, recline on a bed, big chair or sofa, still in view of the mirror. Touch yourself erotically. If you want, do it until you come (and when I say `do it', I mean anything you'd ordinarily do to pleasure yourself). If you're not in the habit of masturbating/self-loving, I'd suggest you read Dr Betty Dodson's wonderful book Sex For One and then come back to this exercise.

• Look at yourself in the mirror - your face as well as your hands and vulva. Watch arousal build. This can be quite erotic - and it is what your chosen voyeur will see if you decide to do this for/with someone else! Take all the time you can spare to do this - thirty minutes is probably a bare minimum if you are going to do the movement and touching exercises all at once. (You can do them separately if you wish.) But longer is better. Among other things, when you add self-pleasuring to this exercise, you are reinforcing yourself with erotic pleasure. The more time you allow, the more you will trust in your own eroticism.

• The next step (which need not happen right away!) is to do this for or with someone else. If it makes you feel braver to have your partner do it along with you, ask him or her to join you. The self-pleasuring part, especially, can be enormously hot for couples to do together. For more suggestions (including what to do if you don't already have an adventuresome partner), see my book *Exhibitionism for the Shy*, which offers practical advice on the fine art of dressing up, showing off, role-playing and talking dirty.

RUTH OSTROW

Permission to be who we already are

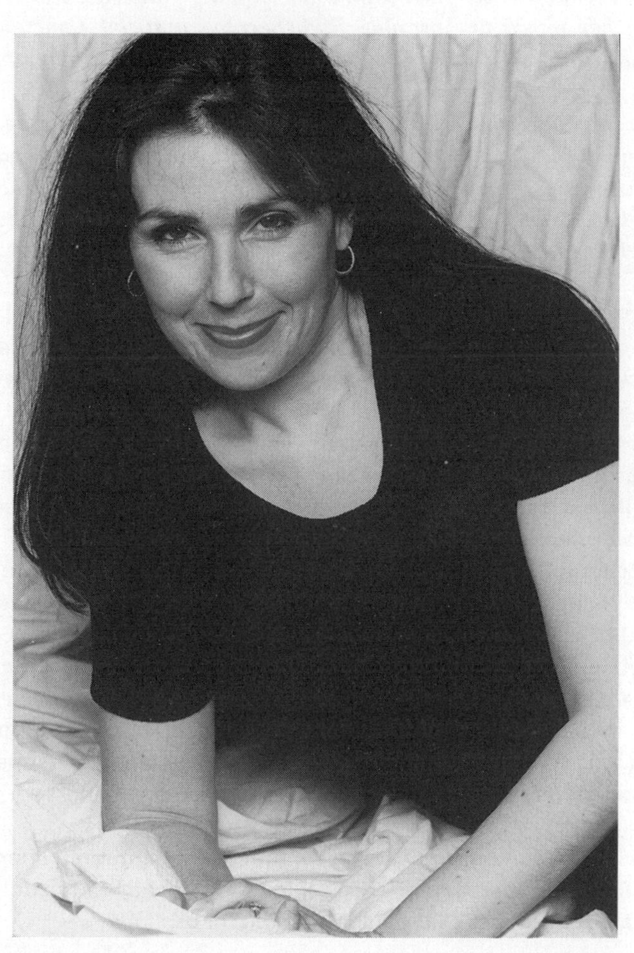

Ruth Ostrow has been a writer and journalist for over fifteen years. During the turbulent 1980s and while working for The Australian Financial Review *she interviewed Australia's top business leaders for her book* The New Boy Network *which revealed the psychology and secrets of success of powerful men, and became a national best-seller.*

After a stint as the Tel Aviv editor of the Israel Economist, *Ruth moved to New York where she witnessed profound changes to the male-dominated corporate culture, which ultimately led her into writing about the men's movement, and finally about the impact the gender revolution was having on male-female relationships.*

On her return to Australia, Ruth became a social commentator, columnist and satirist for The Australian *newspaper, combining her quirky sense of humour with her years of journalistic experience, before she joined the News Limited papers where she now has her own national, weekly page on sexuality and relationships. She also has her own top-rating national radio show. The following extract is adapted from the introduction to* Burning Urges: Australia's Sexual Fantasies *by Ruth Ostrow.*

I remember clearly the experience of going through therapy. I went in a confused and very anxious young woman, and would emerge each week feeling a little better about myself. Despite the tears and the pain that therapy inevitably elicits, each month brought me closer to happiness until I started feeling good, then wonderful, and then as if I could do or be anything I so desired. Eventually, I walked out with such a profound feeling of self-confidence, exuberance and empowerment that the effects have endured a decade later.

Recently I visited my therapist to ask the secret of her success. She explained that her formula was simple. She merely gave me and her other clients permission to be who we already are. She freed us by helping cut away the prescriptions of who we should be, and what we should be doing, thinking and feeling, that had been hung on us by parental desire, peer pressure and social expectation. She allowed us to rejoice and celebrate the essence of our personalities and bodies, and in so doing, allowed us to become the best we could be.

Hers was a message of self-acceptance and liberation: liberation from the deep resentment and self-loathing, disappointment, envy, guilt, fear and regret that plague so many of us.

One thing I carried away from her was a burning desire to take her message to others. She had taught me that I could do and be anything I wanted. What I most wanted to be was a liberator – a person who gave others the same permission she had given me, permission denied to so many by judgemental teachers, parents and various authority figures. Permission to follow your own calling. Permission to be.

This is what motivated me to put together *Burning Urges*, a compilation of people's secret sexual fantasies and inner worlds. In 1996, the News Limited Sunday newspapers across Australia – for whom I work as a journalist – ran 'The Great Australian Sex and Relationships Survey' for me so I could glean statistical information on Australian interpersonal behaviour. In less than three weeks we received just under 10,000 responses.

I was astounded, not only by the revelations buried in the letters but also because so many respondents thanked me for allowing them to express and unburden themselves. Many stated that they had kept all these thoughts 'bottled up' and had felt tormented or guilty about having them. They explained that releasing and sharing them had liberated and excited them.

I decided to see if I could duplicate the success of my earlier inquiries by putting a small advertisement at the bottom of my column in these same newspapers, asking for sexual fantasies for a book. Again, I was immediately swamped with letters. In under two weeks I had received the equivalent of two books full of erotica. And what was revealed was the stunning, strange and bizarre thoughts that lurk in all of our minds. From my largely middle-class readers came a panty-sniffer who fancies old ladies, a happy wife who is obsessed by the idea of exposing her genitals, a happily married man and father who gets sexually aroused imagining a lighted cigarette inserted up his bum. Another gets off fantasising his wife is kidnapped by thugs and gang-banged.

This letter came with a photo of nappies on a clothesline. `Dear Ruth, I am an average, 75-kg Australian male. I do not smoke nor drink alcohol. I have a high-pressure job and, as you see from my photos, I have very different sexual fantasies, which I put into real life. I have high sexual pleasure in wearing nappies and plastic pants at home. It is also a real turn-on to see a partner in her nappy and plastic pants walking around the house... 'Many average, Australian men fantasised about watching their wives go with other men in threesomes, only to reveal later in the fantasy that the la tent wish was to be anally penetrated themselves. Just as many happily married, rugged, outdoorsy Australian men and fathers secretly dressed up in women's clothing, and imagined they were women when having sex: 'My fantasy is to wear nylons, nail polish and high heels while having sex. I love the feel of nylon on my feet, which are about a size seven and are sexy, and to see my nails with pink polish... fuck... it turns me on just writing this!' Such revelations, I believe, help redefine 'normality' and in doing so, allow us more freedom to be.

They confront the way we perceive masculinity. From these admissions we can see that it is impossible to use the beauty stereotype of 'all men desire tall, leggy blondes with large breasts'. In their secret thoughts men desire other men, men dressed as women, fat women, older women, dirty women with sexy smells, horny, raunchy women with body hair and foul mouths. One pensioner, married for decades, craves a large, black, African male in drag. The world of sexual fantasy knows no boundaries and pays little homage to stereotypical aesthetics. And it is certainly free of any hint of political correctness.

Women, too, are a surprising lot. The letters I received were full of happy mothers and wives who want to be consumed by vampires, drink blood and urine, have lesbian mistresses strap them up and torture them to orgasm, take part in lesbian orgies or watch their husbands or partners being screwed by other men. I have always maintained women are as dirty and pornographic as men. It's just that we've been unable to express it. Common wisdom has always maintained that women have romantic fantasies while men's fantasies are more sexual.

As a woman, I have both. My daydreams are very romantic, classic Mills & Boon. They may become sexual, but are more often satiated by a fantasy kiss with some unobtainable *objet d'amour*. I know instinctively that they are about my need for validation and acceptance, probably a bit of escapism in the face of domesticity, and a natural female yearning for high drama that started in our teenage years.

The second type of fantasy I have is the sexual fantasy, which is your garden-variety perverse journey into the undergrowth of the mind. And this is as graphic and pornographic as any male fantasy I have ever read.

So in homage to my therapist, I feel I have put together a work that will ultimately liberate. *Burning Urges* contains material that is a profound challenge to all the acceptable faces we present as mothers, fathers, employees and children. It is not about the side we present that makes society comfortable and complies with the rules, but our most hidden, secret places. Who we are when we dream, when we yearn, when we fear, when we grieve, when we confront death, when we orgasm. It is a book about our pain, our pleasure, our unquenchable appetites and strange lusts. The primal and primitive side of human nature – the rebellious, the perverse, the angry, and untameable side.

It is about the hurt child and the wounded animal who lives beneath the church-going facade. The sexual, sensual, lascivious creature that many conservative thinkers have, for so long, tried to deny. It is about the parts of ourselves that we must learn to love and accept if we are ever to be free.

It is interesting that many conservative thinkers have always told us that only barbaric or warped individuals enjoy watching pornography or have dirty thoughts. And yet the profile of my correspondents belies that. Those riddled with pornographic fantasies are not lonely, isolated, dirty, old men in raincoats or women without love. A large percentage of my respondents are not only married, but happily so. Many have children and share a loving family and religious life together. Many also share their fantasies with their partners as a tool to keep their relationship hot and spicy.

Respected American writer Erica Jong, in her biography *Fear of Fifty*, says her current and third marriage is successful where her other marriages failed for one reason. She has a new habit of writing down her sexual fantasies and reading them to her husband. She claims this is a potent ingredient that helps to preserve sexual arousal and passion in the marriage and enrich communication.

Having grown up with Nancy Friday and now working on my own body of research, I can safely say that none of us is wrong for having our fantasies, no matter how bizarre or questionable. I have long believed that sexual fantasies are gateways to our fears, our motivations, and our childhoods. They are rich in symbolism – and the symbols can be used as a tool to unlock the psyche.

The sexual fantasy, like the dream, is a compilation of subconscious messages and buried feelings. And these fantasies are about far more than sex. They are about what frightens or eludes us, what we crave, or regret, but ultimately – like the sleeping dream – what we need to resolve about our complex lives.

I have always believed that if you understand a person's sexual fantasy, you at once find the key to his or her innermost being. The motivation. The *raison d'être*. You find clues to childhood. The true state of mind. Here are some examples from the letters I received.

'I recall from my teenage years finding it very difficult to get to sleep unless I thought about extreme violence towards women, mostly thrusting a sword into her vagina. I had always been very shy with girls, had an unusually strong-willed mother and an emotionally cold father.

'I have never actually been violent with a partner and cannot think of any reason why I ever would. My strong mother used emotional blackmail as a matter of course to get her own way. I could feel her intense anger very deeply, and experience churning in my solar plexus.'If this doesn't make my point, here is another very telling fantasy from a woman who fantasises about her man and her, in a *ménage-a-trois* with another woman.

'Sometimes I change roles and become the man attending to me or her; then I can change and become her. All parts are interchangeable. This used to trouble me. Was I insecure? Was I jealous? Did my jealousy or envy for the woman translate into pleasure? Was it pain becoming pleasure? Trying to resolve rejection by becoming my rival?' Our fantasies tell us so much and yet they are an under-valued tool by the help professions because analysing them entails the discomforting and thorny issue of sex. In my experience of trying to find a therapist, I found few who wanted to go down this path.

I think it most ironic that sleeping dreams have been elevated to such a lofty status that Jungian dream analysis is almost a science. Yet sexual fantasies – the waking personification – steeped in Oedipal yearnings, unresolved issues and needs, often confound or embarrass many in the help professions.

Thankfully, I found a therapist who paid homage to this inner world. She was not shocked or alarmed by some of the things my mind dug up. She found me neither perverse nor bizarre, rather she used my fantasies to help me unlock the deepest feelings about myself, my parents, my surrounds.

What I discovered was that my head was like a juke-box – full of fantasies waiting to be played. And that I had been using sexual fantasies for years as a way of inadvertently dealing with, or making sense of, my world. If I was feeling a little powerless, I would fantasise about taking control. If I felt over-burdened by power, responsibility and control, I would lapse into a world where power was taken from me, much like the judges and politicians who frequent the SM haunts about town. In short, I was using fantasies almost as a balancing tonic to help me come back to an equilibrium.

And if fantasies are indeed a healing tool or a psychological indicator, a grab for power, a need for validation, then I certainly watched mine change throughout therapy as I struggled to come to terms with many feelings. I saw anger at my parents translate into fantasies concerning authority figures; insecurity led to my waking dreams being filled with 'conquering' imagery. I experienced fantasies about other women as I struggled to love myself, to hatch out my own identity separate from my mother. I yearned to crawl back into the womb and then to break free from it.

After my time on the therapy couch and then putting together *Burning Urges*, I have very much come to see sexual fantasies as a journey into self. A release valve. A medicine of sorts, but best of all, a silent teacher. A teacher directing us to our inner wisdom.

While the wowser element of society has tried to intimidate us into suppressing this healing and self-educational process on the basis that it will lead to aberrant behaviour, many psychologists and researchers I interviewed as part of my research now confirm that fantasies are not necessarily things we want to do. Often, they are just the opposite. For many they are simply a cathartic experience that can be mentally rejected the moment after orgasm.

For instance, many women have rape or abuse fantasies for a variety of reasons. But in such a fantasy, the fantasiser remains in control, the one to turn off the images at whim, change events, increase or decrease the tension. A woman can play out a past trauma, her worst fears or most forbidden yearnings, yet she can stop the fantasy, redress the balance, play either role and identify with either party to quell her anxiety. She has the control button.

One of the most curative effects of fantasies are that they allow us to explore different roles, obsessions or fixations with impunity and in the safety of our own heads. We are empowered by our own ability to direct and command events?so rare in real life and in the murky waters of interpersonal relationships.

Even better, fantasies lead us to such explosive and marvellous orgasms, with a partner or alone! There is one more fantastic benefit, not to be overlooked. Sexual fantasies are the ultimate safe sex.

KIMBERLY O'SULLIVAN

A warrior with words

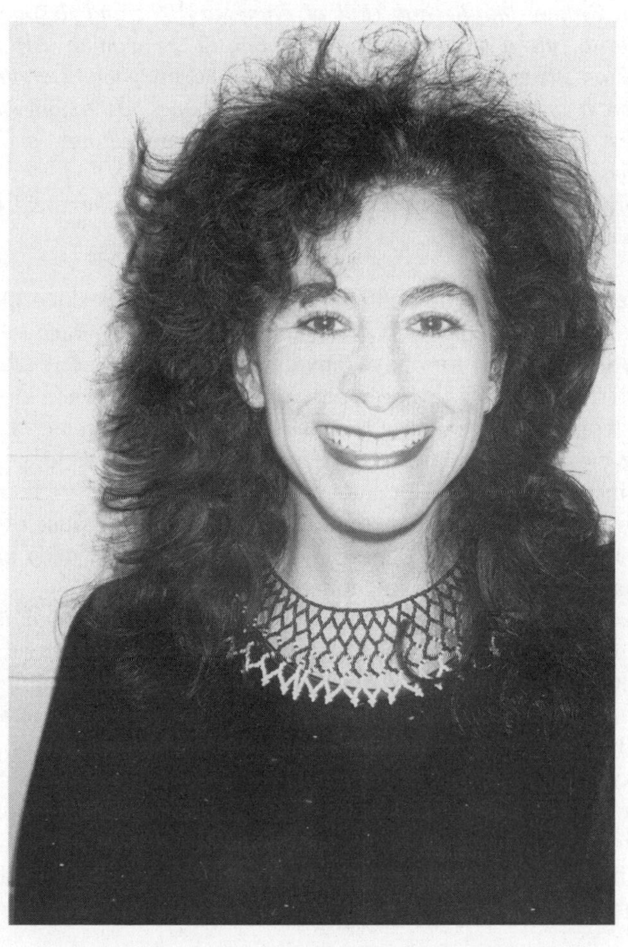

Kimberly O'Sullivan is a social justice activist. She has worked in the Left, the union movement, the women's movement and for gay and lesbian liberation. She is most well-known for her sexual libertarian views, public speaking, hands-on sex toy workshops for women and extensive writing on sexual hypocrisy, sexual freedom and the sexual empowerment of women. She has been published widely in the alternative, sex and mainstream press. Her work has appeared in anthologies and she has had her own radio show and been a university guest lecturer.

For two years Kimberly was the editor of Wicked Women, *Australia's only lesbian sex magazine. She was the first woman elected to the Sydney Mardi Gras Hall of Fame in 1992 and despite being unable to ride a motorbike, she was one of the women who started Dykes on Bikes. A journalist and editor of twenty years' standing, she is also a qualified archivist and historian and has a long-standing interest in the hidden history of cultural minority groups and erotic outlaws. Kimberley's life has taken her in a new direction - she is now celebrating her sexuality and passion for life with her new (male) husband.*

I have been writing and politically agitating about sex since 1985 and it has affected my life in ways I could never have imagined. It has done great things for me. I have had amazing experiences, met wonderful (and bizarre) people who have given me a depth of knowledge about sexuality that most people only dream of. It has made me a more compassionate person, certainly less judgemental and increasingly it has made me see sexuality as an incredibly precious gift. I have seen people's lives destroyed because of sexual secrets and oppression, and I have seen people heal deep parts of themselves through sexual connection.

Along the way I have had every sort of sex I ever wanted, fulfilled most of my sexual fantasies and had some toecurling nights that will take me to my grave with a smile on my face. I have also endured the frustration of lesbian bed death (the cessation of sexual relations), raged at selfish, inconsiderate lovers, ached at the pain of sexual betrayal and rejection, and cried buckets of tears over a broken heart. I've learned along the way that it all goes with the erotic territory. And maybe my passionate personality.

The strangest thing about my life is that I never wanted to be controversial, notorious or in the public eye and somehow I have managed all three. I wanted to tell the truth, I wanted to expose lies and in the beginning I naively thought that this would make me seem courageous, maybe even honourable.

I started writing in the area of sexuality by accident. I was formerly a book reviewer, but always had an abiding interest and (seemingly) limitless curiosity about sexuality. When I read about other sexuality writers we all seem to have this curiosity about sex and acknowledge that this is where people keep their deepest, darkest secrets. I had a desire to dig down and find out what they were hiding and why they were being hidden in their sexuality.

As a writer I have always lived by Dorothy Allison's belief that writers have to tell the truth, otherwise they are writing lies. I used to have that quote stuck above the desk where I wrote. I put it there to remind me to be courageous. I started to turn that vision for truth, that curiosity toward the women I knew, the women I had sex with, the gay men I hung out with and the men I met through the sex industry.

So I started to write and research and found an eager market in the emerging gay publications and regular readers whose support convinced editors to keep publishing my (then) off-the-wall views on sex and sexuality. When I was still considered too 'controversial' for lesbian magazines, it was gay male magazines that supported my work and allowed me to publish the first Australian articles on the feminist sex wars and the emerging lesbian SM scene.

Sometimes I still don't see what I did or wrote that was so outrageous, because I based the columns and articles I used to write about female sexuality and, specifically lesbian sexual culture, on the stories of the women around me and what I was doing with my lovers. I didn't make it up, although my detractors often accused me of making up sensational lies to either (a) advance my own career or (b) shock and disturb the equilibrium of the gay girl world.

When I wrote about SM it was because we were doing it. When I wrote about discovering my femme identity, loving butches and playing with gender it was because I was doing it and so were the women around me. It came as a great shock then to be regularly pilloried because of my outrageous views, to have acquaintances refuse to acknowledge me in public lesbian venues and to have editors nervously treble-checking my articles for something that might offend readers.

When I started writing about the sex industry it was as an

insider. Like the other areas I explored it was as a participant, not a voyeur. It was an area where I felt the weight of lies and the damage that stereotypes do add another layer of oppression on women who make their living in the adult industry.

I see myself as a warrior with words, a sexual scribe. Words are my weapons and where the power of my influence lies. I've been writing since I could hold a pencil and cannot envisage a time when I will stop. But fifteen years down the track I am now doing a lot of reassessing. I took a ten-year journey through the SM world, but it is now not somewhere that I choose to live. I will always be a femme, but not necessarily in relation to a butch. My sexual identity is much more fluid than before. I now don't want to expose my life, relationships and friends in print; I feel the need for privacy and reflection more than candid exposure in the name of getting at the truth.

TIPS FOR SAFER SEX IN THE WORLD

- Write a letter to your local MP today about a sexual issue in your electorate. Are the police harassing sex workers? Is your local adult shop under attack?

- At a dinner party bring up the topic of sexual rights and responsibilities and get people in a heated debate.
Abortion is sexual freedom of choice. Remember to make the link to friends and colleagues.

- Homophobia is sexual repression. Say so at every opportunity.

- Don't let anyone get away with jokes about sex workers or sexual violence toward women (so-called `rape' jokes). These are both based on sexual hatred.

- Do something sexually joyful for yourself every week - flirt with a stranger, wear something extra special and sexy to bed (no excuses just because you are sleeping alone) and think up a new potent sexual fantasy (don't just rely on the old ones).

- Remember the three Ms: massage, masturbation and meditation, and make them a regular part of your life.

What still remains important is to speak up about political sexual repression.

5

Physical Challenges

In an era where discussion of sexuality is supposedly open and without limits there is a significant number of women whose sexual issues are not only not on the agenda for discussion, but whose sexuality is almost seen as taboo. These are women who are aging, facing physical challenges or ill health. In the late twentieth century sexuality is portrayed as an activity for the beautiful, young and physically 'perfect'. This is particularly reinforced in film, where the Hollywood erotic ideal and gymnastic sexuality dominate, which few people can live up to even if they wanted. In the celluloid world people are easily orgasmic, always satisfied and 'ugly' bodily fluids never spoil a beautiful erotic moment.

The perception of perfect bodies, perfect sex and multiple orgasms excludes a large percentage of the human race whose sexuality is often complicated, less than satisfactory and beset by physical and emotional contradictions. Perpetuating only a limited range of what is the acceptable face of sexuality leaves the large percentage of women who are post-menopausal, physically challenged or living with a life-threatening illness with few places to go for an alternative view.

Although they are traditionally viewed as 'sexless', these women often have a personal sexual expression that is a source of joy and physical delight. In their triumphant sexuality they defy Hollywood-imposed stereotypes, yet they are still not positively represented in public depictions of the sexually active.

Aging

Once, pregnancy was viewed as a 'sickness', with pregnant women seen as unsexual, unsexy and hiding their big bellies under tent-like maternity clothes. This view has changed as gutsy pregnant women rebelled and started to demand that they be seen as not only normal, but healthy. When celebrities, such as Demi Moore, did nude pregnant photo spreads, the view of the pregnant body permanently altered.

The same revolution for post-menopausal women is still to happen. Menopause is only just coming off the 'not to be discussed in public' list, but it is seen in many quarters as an illness, and not a normal, inevitable part of every woman's life. As the baby-boomer generation hits menopause this view is being transformed and the same women who said 'pregnancy is not an illness' are now saying 'and neither is menopause'.

However, images in popular culture do not reflect this, and older women still have to struggle with outmoded stereotypes that equate female beauty with youthfulness. The more this happens the more older women are disempowered and not viewed as beautiful. In those cultures where women's power and status are not tied to youthfulness, their value to society increases as they age.

Ancient cultures which revered the triple goddess, whose manifestations are maid, mother and crone, gave equal value to each of these stages of every woman's life. When a woman reached her crone stage she was seen as wise, with the knowledge of a lifetime at her fingertips. Her aging skin, white hair and gnarled fingers were seen to have their own unique beauty. It is rare in Western culture today to see an older woman who looks like this described as beautiful, even rarer for her to be described as sexual.

Physical challenges

The physically challenged have the same right as able-bodied people to a sexual expression they deem is appropriate. Their situation often means they need an understanding carer who is able to act on their behalf – for example to purchase sex toys or to arrange a sex surrogate. Carers themselves may fear that intervention on their clients' behalf could be misinterpreted as inappropriate sexual behaviour, and so may be reluctant to advocate for their clients in this area. However, carers are frequently family members or a parent – to negotiate the role of a sexually active adult with one's parent is frequently embarrassing.

While the traditional role of the church in running institutions and other facilities for the physically challenged have been beneficial, it has often been at the cost of ignoring the sexual needs and rights of these people. This is not just based on religious dogma or sexual intolerance; carers in such institutions may share the embarrassment of the wider community when confronted by the sexuality of people with disabilities.

Because it is difficult for people with disabilities to meet sexual partners their ability to explore their own sexuality is limited. Their opportunities for spontaneous sex are restricted by the necessity to negotiate wheelchairs, catheters and colostomy bags. The partners of physically challenged people need sensitivity and patience, and where both partners are physically challenged their intimate life may require the intervention of their carers.

A view of sexuality that says it is for the physically perfect by its definition excludes anyone who lives daily with muscle spasms, limited movement and speech difficulties. Such a limited view is not only ignorant but can cruelly affect the sexual self-esteem of people living with physical challenges.

Illness

Those who suffer from chronic or life-threatening illness often find ways to keep their sexuality alive. Many people facing serious illness see their sexuality as a connection to the lifeforce. Yet sick people are never seen as sexual; to view them this way is even regarded as obscene.

There is a way to strike a balance between looking after someone and still allow him or her the dignity of sexual expression. While no-one should be coerced into a sexual situation when ill, if someone requests intimate time with his or her partner, this should not be viewed as abhorrent.

Sexuality can manifest in lots of different ways, not just heterosexual, penetrative sex. Erotic touch and massage can be a healing, affirmative expression of love and a healing moment for someone feeling disconnected from their body when dealing with illness. To be touched is to feel loved, and from childhood to when we die, this does not change. A massage service set up for people living with HIV/AIDS has reported wonderful feedback from people to massage, even when they have been in great pain or in the terminal stages of this disease.

In this chapter the personal experiences of Joan Nestle, the work of Tuppy Owens and Rosie King illuminate the connection between the body, illness, aging, physical challenges and being sexually alive.

JOAN NESTLE

Let my desire remain

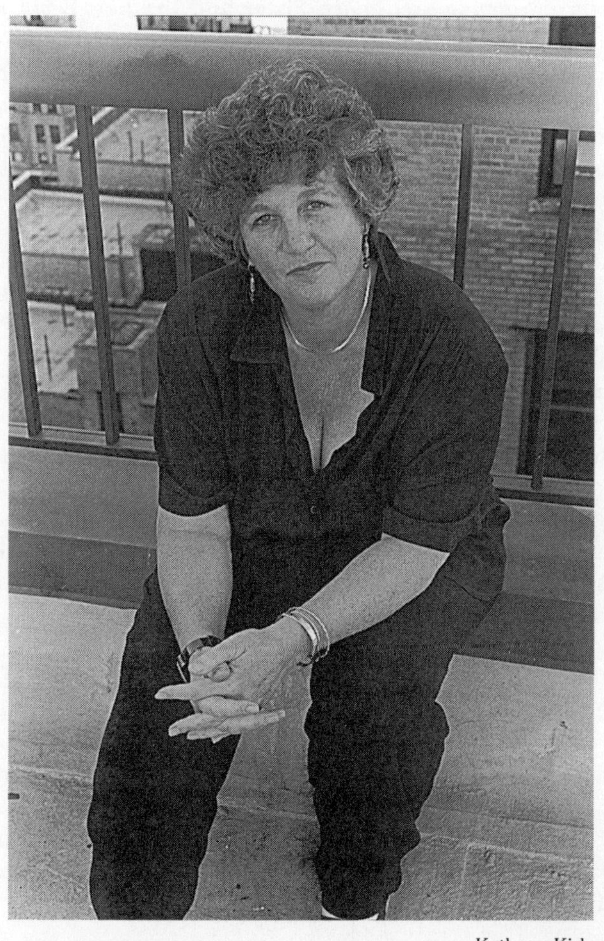

Kathryn Kirk

Joan Nestle was born in New York City in 1940, a working-class Jew raised by her mother who worked as a bookkeeper in the garment industry. She came out as lesbian in Greenwich Village in the 1950s, marched in Selma in 1965, joined the ranks of the feminist movement in 1971, and helped establish the Gay Academic Union in 1972. In 1973, Joan co-founded the Lesbian Herstory Archives, which now fills a three-storey building in Park Slope, Brooklyn.

Joan is the author of A Restricted Country *and editor of* The Persistent Desire: A Femme-Butch Reader. *She is co-editor (with Naomi Holoch) of* Worlds Unspoken: An Anthology of International Lesbian Fiction *and the 'Women on Women' lesbian fiction series. With John Preston, she co-edited* Sister and Brother: Lesbians and Gay Men Write About Their Lives Together.

She has won numerous awards, including the Bill Whitehead Award for Lifetime Achievement in Lesbian and Gay Literature, the America Library Association Gay/Lesbian Book Award and the Lambda Literary Award for Lesbian Nonfiction. She lives in New York.

The following is an extract from Joan Nestle's book, A Fragile Union, *published by Cleis Press, San Francisco, 1998.*

15 January 1997

I haven't been able to write a word since I was told I have colon cancer. All of it – the bleeding, the tests, the operation, the chemo, the fissure that will not heal, and the doctors who did everything so fast and did not listen to me – all now embody everything I detest, including my own body. Embody. I embody disease and disavowal, blood and shit and a body bound in pain. Everything tastes like acid now, like car batteries in my mouth. If ever words could bring me life, and they have, please, please do it now.

The ex-lover

She stands, so fresh and open, in the doorway, a gray scarf hung loosely from her muscled neck. Her green winter jacket is already zipped, and in her right hand is a large blue carry-all, bulging with tools. I turn to say good-bye and all time stops. This woman with whom I have shared a decade as lovers.

This woman who sat by my bed in a darkened hospital room, hour after hour, keeping guard. One night in the hazy but impenetrable sleep of drugs, I felt someone tug at my fingers and thought it was the nurse taking my blood, but it was my love gently sliding back onto my finger the ring she had given me ten years ago, before the flood of cells.

The reading: February 1998

A year after my surgery, I was asked to participate in a reading from a new collection of lesbian erotica. The editor had selected my story 'A Different Place', a story written in 1986, that celebrated the pleasure of anal fucking. This was my first public appearance as a writer since the cancer, and up to the last minute I did not know if I would be able to read that story in public. Everyone before me read from their piece that appeared in the collection. When I stepped up to the microphone, I thought I would give it a try, but as I read the opening passages of the story, describing the preparation Jay was going through to be ready to perform anal penetration, I knew that I would stop before the scene of entry.

I have colon-rectal cancer and it may kill me, that story overwhelmed the narrative of a night of pleasure in Connecticut over ten years ago. Torn between still wanting to preserve the space I had opened for my audience, the space that allowed women to enjoy all forms of sexual activity, and my own recent need for sexual silence, I chose as gracefully as I could to leave them with the sense of wonderful expectation, the promise that the story would bring them pleasure – but I could not go there with them, I explained, because of my cancer.

My body

This is now my battle, to win back from the specifics of medical treatment – from the outrage of an invaded body where hands I did not know touched parts of myself that I will never see – my own body, my own body so marked by the hands and lips of lovers, now so lonely in its fear. Touch my scar, knead my belly, don't be afraid of my cancer. Enter me the old way, not through the skin cut open, but because I am calling to you through the movement of my hips, the breath that pleads for your hand to touch the want of me. Heal me because you do not fear me, touch me because you do not fear the future. Cancer and sex. One I have and one I must have.

The new lover

Like a little girl bringing out a favourite doll, I shouted from the bedroom, 'I need to show you something.' You, my new friend, were sitting at the dining-room table and turned expectantly toward me when I reappeared. 'I need you to see this,' I said, holding up my shirt and pulling down the band of my pants so you could see the still-red scar that started at my waist, skirted my belly button, and made its way down to the beginning of my pubic triangle.

I stood in front of you, not clear about why I was doing this, a fifty-seven-year-old woman exhibiting her cancer scar to a new friend. You reached out and traced the path of the incision with your fingers, and I started to cry. Not a little girl any more, but a woman with colon cancer, a cancer that should have been found when I had the colonoscopy done a year before the tumour grew so large it invaded the surrounding tissue, but that a rushed doctor had missed.

'I pulled out too quickly,' he told me later, after the tumour had broken through the wall of my colon and spilled red blood into the toilet bowl. 'Have you cried yet?' he asked me in 1997. It took a year for the tears to come, and they came only when I stood in front of a woman whom I wanted to touch me, to make love to me like it used to be.

My treatment

It will never be like it used to be. Cancer has claimed me; 'my cancer', I say now, like others talk about their cars or children. We suggest you have a year of chemo, the doctors said, and I did – or as much of it as I could stand. For that whole year, I did not allow anyone to touch me, except doctors, nurses, technicians. My body was filled with chemicals that sickened me. I sat on the edges of tables in small cubicles, the IV needle precariously housed in my arm, in a small vein on the back of my hand or anywhere else the oncologist could find a vein large enough and strong enough to absorb the needle and the acid. Sometimes the vein would collapse, and the chemo would start pouring out under my skin. 'You are lucky,' the doctor said. 'This chemo is not as dangerous as some of the others. 'And I knew he was right, I was one of the 'lucky' ones. I would keep my hair, I avoided a shunt; I only had 500 mg of 5-FU every week with 50 mg of Leucovorin, a form of folic acid, a natural substance that some people want to ingest. I had not been able to take the initial treatment, 5-FU with Ergamisole, a drug used to kill worms in the stomachs of sheep. After two treatments with the little white pills, I did not care if I lived or died.

This is not the story of every cancer patient; it is my own, just like this cancer, this colon rectal cancer, is my own. Just like this body, now a year and a half after the surgeon removed four feet of colon, my transverse colon, and reattached my intestines in a new configuration, is my own. I need you to know all the details, the scientific names, the side-effects, just as I had to learn them. Illness, like sex, gives the body another dimension, makes it transparent. I could feel the chemotherapy liquid enter my veins, trace its burning journey through my arm, just as I used to feel a lover's tongue trail down my neck.

Like so many others, I am caught in the limbo of cancer, the still place at the heart of the night. I cannot travel back to the physical safety I once thought I had, and I cannot go forward with any assurances that I have a future. I am not unique in this stasis, but this is my bedroom, my history; these are my questions of endurance. How will I travel in my life? What belongings will I carry with me?Let my desire remain, even if the cancer grows again into its grey mounds of life. Let my breasts and cunt grow hard with answering determination. And let me keep what I have learned from this illness – that terror is a human thing, that the body, even in its vomit and blood, wants to stand on its feet again, that kindness makes its way through the dead skin, that sickness, too, yearns for its human voice. These are my travels. Late in the night, I will go deep into my body's story and hear its tale of life battling life. And as I welcomed home my other beloved travellers, I will bury my head in the gift of hope only I can bring to the surface.

TUPPY OWENS

With a healthy sex life

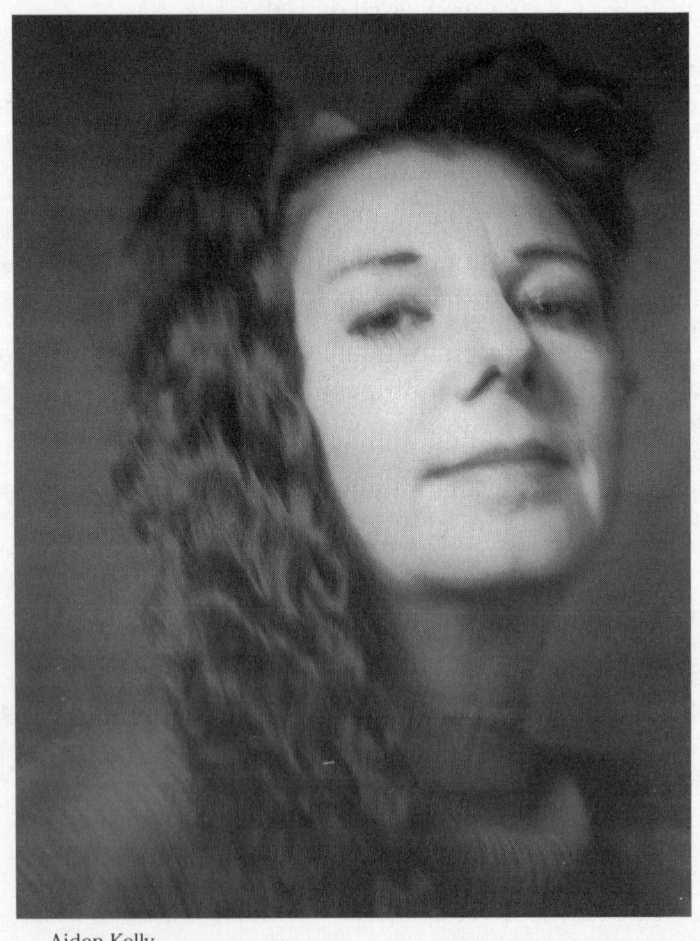

Aiden Kelly

Tuppy Owens has a Diploma in Human Sexuality from London University and an honorary doctorate for her 'good works'. Born in Cambridge, UK, she was the second child of a tertiary-educated man from a well-to-do background and a local girl from a working-class family. Her father was known for his dirty jokes, so she grew up learning that sex was funny. While her father let her do as she wanted, when her mother discovered a letter Tuppy had written about trying to have sex with a man she was ordered straight off to Sunday school.

When she was seventeen, she travelled to the Serengeti to join her boyfriend counting wildebeest. When she returned to London she read Zoology at Exeter, whizzed away to Trinidad and eventually ended up in London, where she discovered pornography on her boyfriend's father's printing press. It was to change her life.

I felt pornographic magazines were an insult to sex, so I rushed away to take some better photos and design better books. I was amazed when told that the self-portraits I'd taken on a riverbank at dawn with a doll up me were illegal. I accepted the restrictions and went on to produce a very happy book that kept within the law, called *Sexual Harmony*. It included pretty photos of a charming couple in lots of exciting sex positions, and my attempts to explain how to fuck and have fun.

What I had done for free as a challenge became a nice little earner, and the books sold a hundred copies a week in a new London sex shop. This financed other photo shoots and soon I was producing a series, *Love in the Open Air*, with pics taken in the British countryside of couples copulating, in spring, summer, autumn and winter. My writing gained confidence and became quite tender and poetic.

One Christmas a gay couple came to stay from Amsterdam and, on departing, promised to send me a saucy Dutch diary as a thank-you gift. Halfway into January, it still hadn't arrived (there was probably no such thing) and I began to fantasise about turning the pages of a dated scrapbook to discover a lovely porno pic in front of my eyes every morning of the year. The idea grew, and I thought I'd produce a *Sex Maniac's Diary* to mimic the other hobbyist diaries of the era, giving facts and figures, all presented formally. As well as a great joke I liked the idea of treating sex with the same respect and detail as other pastimes.

The 1973 *Sex Maniac's Diary* came out on 12 December 1972 and sold out in two weeks. I carried on producing this little book for twenty-three years. At its peak, it was selling over 100,000 copies a year. *The Diary* gave me the chance to research what was going on in the swing and fetish scene and many other scenes all over the world, so I became something of an international expert. Clubs and hotels were reviewed but were also allocated symbols, denoting certain erotic characteristics and qualities. When AIDS hit, I reviewed condoms and drew pictures from Polaroids I'd shot of me and my then-favourite cock of how to put on a condom. I changed the name to the *Safer Sex Maniac's Diary*.

I took great pride and worked very hard to produce each issue. By the time the *Diary* was established, I had made friends with Annie Sprinkle and a few other pioneers around the world, and we took pleasure in each other's existence. Distributors often tried to censor the *Diary*, as I listed very extreme clubs and groups, but I always found a way to carry on, including the bizarre things, simply by using language the distributors wouldn't understand. I eventually compiled a book called *Planet Sex – The Handbook*, with loads of info in it and dumped the *Diary* for good in 1995.

Producing one annual a year gave me some spare time. In 1978 I met a couple of disabled people who had no social or sexual lives, and helped them remedy that, and thought there must be lots of other isolated people who, with a little reassurance and a few introductions, could have their lives transformed. With a healthy sex life, the disability, pain and disfigurement might even feel less troublesome.

I started Outsiders in 1979. It was run from my home and after a couple of newspaper articles we got lots of fabulous members and held parties, lunches and discussions. We compiled a book called *Practical Suggestions*, published a list of members and a magazine, and it was all tremendous fun. Then the residents of my block objected to my working from home and I was faced with having to rent an office. So I began the Sex Maniac's Ball to raise funds.

Outsiders now has a bright, wheelchair-accessible office in Holland Park, is run by a small band of loyal disabled members, has a management committee of members with varied disabilities, and is going from strength to strength. This isn't to say we haven't had problems – these have come mostly from the more radical disabled world, where they see self-help groups for disabled people run by so-called able-bodied people, let alone someone involved in pornography, as suspect. Little did they know that just before I began Outsiders, I'd broken up with a boyfriend and found myself totally isolated, and suffering panic attacks.

Being a woman sex writer and self-employed publisher, especially in sex, was isolating. The Club also got attacked by the gutter press, which made up a story linking whores, Lords and disability. We have never really recovered. Some members told me that before coming to an Outsiders event, people in their residential homes teased them about their forthcoming orgy – a painful experience if you're still a virgin and desperate to find a loving partner.

Even today, some radical disability activists say that any relationship between a disabled person and an able-bodied person must be exploitative. I know differently. One of our first couplings was between a girl with mild learning difficulties and a chemistry teacher with acne. Very happy they were too. I remember a blind girl asking her father what he thought of her new boyfriend and Dad complained that he was black – news to the blind girl – but she didn't care! We accept everyone for what they are, so long as they don't express prejudice of any kind. We acknowledge their sexuality, however disabled or disfigured. I wish we had more success but don't you all wish for more of that too! We always have too many men and not enough women. The women are put off by our sexy reputation, and are often incredibly timid. On top of which, it's easier for disabled women to find partners in a society where men want someone to have sex with and marry and women feel they should have a partner their parents and friends will approve of.

Many of the men complain bitterly of sexual frustration while few of the women do. We've had to be careful of introducing the men to prostitutes because we could get done for pimping. Anyway, most prostitutes don't use their time with the men to educate and teach them, they just provide an easy (and enjoyable) screw or fantasy experience which does little to help the chap go out and find a real relationship. I'd like to train surrogates but will have to wait until our laws are reformed.

Soon after I'd started Outsiders, I decided to take a course in sex therapy and was delighted to get into a two-year post-doctorate course at a London hospital as part of London University. This gave me loads of confidence and the capacity to answer members' questions with more knowledge. I got invited to talk about the club at conferences and it seemed that people were far more impressed in foreign countries. Back home, people still preferred to attack me.

While I was touring America doing research for the *Sex Maniac's Diary*, I was meeting dozens of really interesting sexual adventurers, running clubs and doing things, but none of them ever met each other. I decided to put on an international erotic event, and realised it could also raise funds for Outsiders. Rather like Robin Hood – using those who have plenty to provide for those who have none.

The first ball was in 1986 and it was wild. I had no idea how to run a club or large party but we got over 1000 people from all over the world and definitely did not get invited back to the venue (The London Dungeon). I am now about to embark on the fourteenth annual event and, once again, have yet to find a venue.

I encourage disabled people to come, swingers, fetishists and boogiers, but most of all, I encourage people with minority tastes who have never expressed them in public before so they can be 'out' and others can meet and accept them. Most of the resulting sideshows and spectacles raise a bit of cash for Outsiders besides providing fun and entertainment but keeping all these revellers responsibly in charge of their collection boxes is a job and a half! The ball has kept going during the entire rise and fall of the fetish scene in London, the dearth of swing clubs swelling up as swingers get used to condoms, and the fascination of youth with experimentation. I have to keep my eye on the moment and create a ball each year that will attract the people despite the ebb and flow of fashion and trend.

Having visited so many sex clubs around the world, I had a wealth of creativity to set me up and we have a fabulous Grope Box, based on an idea I discovered at the swing club Sea Breeze in Marina Del Rey, California. Thank you, Tom! I have still yet to recreate your fabulous Infinity Room, lined with millions of tiny mirrors.

One of my inventions is the Rubber Wall – a large sheet of translucent back-lit rubber, which you can dance or gyrate against and enjoy unknown bodies on the other side. The last ball had a Spanish theme to make everyone feel up and happy, and a troupe of girls did a flamenco dance on top of a fetishist who likes being trampled. Ole! Five years ago, I decided that there's not enough acclaim for people in the sex industry and erotic world who rebel or excel. So I started the Erotic Oscars. This has been a really hard job.

A fabulous team of judges discusses nominations, who shall become finalists and who will actually win the twelve categories, which include sex worker, film and innovator. We put on a stunning exhibition and the finalists who are performers do a show at the Sex

TIPS FOR PHYSICALLY CHALLENGED PEOPLE

The Outsiders have produced a book, *Practical Suggestions*, which lists ways in which physically challenged people have found it easier to date, chat up, seduce someone and have sex. We believe physically challenged people are sexual, and the only way your friends will agree is if you talk about sex, expressing your frustrations and requesting help if you need it.

- Masturbate if you don't have a partner and, if you can't, tell everyone and someone, a sex angel, might come along to do it for you.

- Don't allow people to fob you off with the notion that masturbation is enough. Everyone wants intimacy and you need it just as much as the next person.

- Don't be sexually timid. You only live once. Go out to get rejected and you may be pleasantly surprised. Otherwise you can go home and have a laugh with your friends.

- If people pity you, then pity them, for they don't know you very well, and haven't bothered to discover how great you are.

- A dear friend of mine told me that physically challenged people make the best lovers because they have to think and plan the experience. Spread the word.

Maniac's Ball.

One of the reasons for doing the Oscars is to give the winners positive publicity but, guess what? The press always blank us. It's odd, isn't it? Magazines, newspapers and TV are chock-a-block with sex, but they still want to portray the seamy side and ignore the innovators and people who are really doing good things. Last year, we had the Oscars filmed by the BBC so perhaps we'll get a higher profile in the future.

By the tenth anniversary of the Sex Maniac's Ball, I was beginning to feel confident that it would be socially acceptable. I booked a prestigious venue, designed a really exotic and rude flier, had loads of new ideas and was ready for a big splash. Perhaps it had something to do with the British Government finally making anal sex legal and I'd called the venue on the flier 'The Anal Academy' or perhaps we were too high profile but anyway, the cops decided to stop the event, so 1500 people, some of whom had flown in from as far as Tokyo, arrived at an empty building, while I was trying to give the £8000 worth of food prepared for the guests to London's homeless. I'd had so many setbacks before in my life, I took it all in my stride.

The Outsiders was broke, but we had been broke before. But other people were not amused and, after a public meeting, a march to the Prime Minister was organised, and the Sexual Freedom Coalition was launched. This is a pansexual, non party-political campaign for the sexual freedom of all consenting adults, concerned with law reform, responsible reporting of sex in the media, and educating and encouraging people to enjoy their sexuality to the full. I also edit the campaign newspaper, *Consenting Adults*.

ROSIE KING
Quenching skin hunger

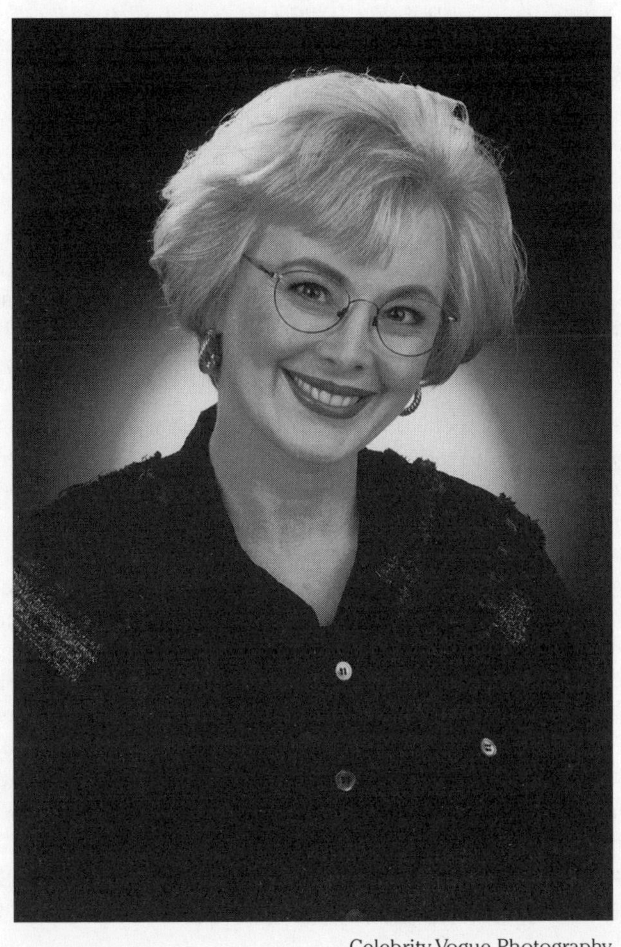

Celebrity Vogue Photography

Rosie King is a doctor with a difference. A sex therapist and sex educator, she has worked consistently in the Australian media for over a decade. Her weekly column in Woman's Day *and regular appearances on television's the* Midday Show *have helped to bring her warmth, humour and sound advice into millions of Australian homes. She is a highly respected regular contributor to The* Australian *newspaper.*

Rosie trained as a medical practitioner at the University of New South Wales and spent ten years in general practice. She is an honorary Fellow of the Australasian College of Sexual Health Physicians and a visiting lecturer at the University of New South Wales in the School of Obstetrics and Gynaecology. She also lectures in the Master of Medicine and Master of Public Health degrees at the University of Sydney. She is the author of a best-selling book, Good Loving, Great Sex.

Having worked in the area of sexuality for many years I recognise that I have the same fears, anxieties and worries as everyone else. Because I recognise that I am not immune to these has given me a natural kindness when I work in this area. Kindness in this sense means that I feel 'of a kind', part of the herd; I feel a sense of belonging. This reduces my sense of isolation and stops a feeling of disconnection, because I realise that we all have the same anxieties and worries.

When I was younger I used to think that the people who seemed very emotionally 'together' didn't have any problems, whereas I used to spend all my time focusing on solving my problems. I developed Rosie's theory, which says that no matter how much time I spent trying to solve my problems there were always more to take their place. I decided that life contains a constant stream of problems and although it is a good idea to problem-solve, it cannot be the focus of living.

Since this, my focus has been more on making sure that there are more 'goodies' in my life. My theory says that one 'goodie' equals 100 problems and that happiness comes from not solving problems, but from finding 'goodies'. For me 'goodies' are having sex, walking my dogs, listening to music, spending time with my children, sleeping and eating.

The key to happiness is not being problem-free, it is dealing with your problems and making sure that there are lots of 'goodies' in your life. That is where sex fits in. Sadly, for many people, sex is a source of disappointment, despair, frustration, anxiety and pain. I keep working in this area because I would like sex to be a 'goodie' for everyone.

Every day I accept and value my own sexuality more. I believe if ever you wanted proof that there is a God, you only have to look at the beauty of our sexuality to be convinced, because it is so perfect. I never get sick of talking, learning, thinking or working about sex because I believe our sexuality is a miracle. Desire waxes and wanes naturally throughout our life, but you don't need desire to enjoy sex.

Desire is affected by hormonal problems, physical illness, relationship difficulties and the stresses of everyday life. However, given the right conditions, it is possible to become aroused and enjoy sex without any desire at all. Desire and arousal are two separate components and are run by different parts of the brain. Of course, it is much easier to be turned on if you have a high level of desire. However, sometimes you can be initially sexually disinterested, but if your partner helps to warm you up then often you can have a very pleasurable sexual experience, which can lead to high levels of arousal and orgasm.

There are many times when women feel sexual, but don't feel like penetrative intercourse. However, they might be quite happy to participate in sexual activity that is less demanding. It is important to realise that it is part of the give and take of a long-term relationship.

Often partners need to negotiate a compromise, for example, with a heterosexual couple he might have a need for sex and she may need to be sexually inactive. You can experience physical and emotional closeness without having penetrative sex. This is where 'outercourse' comes in very handy, expanding your concept of what lovemaking is, so that you can make love to your partner and not necessarily get turned on.

Desire is not the only reason for sex – it is an expression of love and affection, fun, pleasure given and received, passion, sensuality, communication, intimacy, procreation, sexual release, tension release, affirmation of desirability, security, confirmation of the relationship, affirmation of gender, nurturing, comfort, to get to sleep, to please your partner or to quench 'skin hunger'. 'Skin hunger', rather than sex drive, is the greatest motivator for sexual contact, and a lot of casual sex is motivated by the need to be touched. This is a basic human need that is present from the time we are born. In the early twentieth century, studies were done in an orphanage on different levels of contact. Babies were separated into two groups: one was fed, bathed and put back to bed, while the other was also cuddled. The group that received minimal touch became sick more often, failed to thrive and had a higher mortality rate. The need to be touched doesn't stop because we reach purity or fifty, it is an important part of being part of being human. We are herd animals, like dogs or horses, and we need skin-on-skin contact and touching for good general health.

In order to continue to make love throughout life we have to ask ourselves what lovemaking is. Is it penis-vagina intercourse? It is not for gay people, and they are much more flexible in their concept of what sex is. Lovemaking is a physical and emotional connection between two people that need not include desire, arousal, erection, lubrication, orgasm or ejaculation. To express our sexuality to the fullest we have to let go of rigid ideas about what constitutes lovemaking. There are many people who, for all sorts of reasons, can't have sexual intercourse.

Judaeo-Christian tradition holds that sex is only for reproduction, which is penetrative sex, but I believe we are far beyond that. It is the difference between making love and copulation. Copulation is for reproductive sex while lovemaking is a much higher, spiritual, emotional and physical connection. Sex is more than passing sperm to eggs.

We should be careful not to lay down guidelines of sexual behaviour for women at certain times of life, such as after childbirth, menopause or following an illness. These are common times for sexual desire to decrease in intensity. Interestingly, humans are the only animals that mate when the females are pregnant or after menopause.

Every woman is an individual and it is true that some women do feel less sexual around childbirth, and in the early months of child-rearing. It also might be that society doesn't see pregnant women as being sexual – they are either 'mothers' or 'whores', not both. For some women it can take years for their sexual response to come back. Some women feel sexy no matter what happens in their life, while for others their sexuality waxes and wanes.

There has always been a bit of shame associated with pregnancy, with the pregnant body hidden in voluminous maternity clothes, instead of close-fitting ones. Western society tends to desexualise pregnant women, which is fine for some women, but not for others who feel very alive and sexual. I had one patient who told me that during her pregnancy she felt like an Earth Goddess, the fountain of all living things.

Ill women certainly aren't seen as sexy. When someone assumes the patient's role, they become stripped of their identity, power and status. There is often a patronising approach to patients, which leads to the person feeling disempowered and asexual. The patient becomes 'the breast cancer in bed 24' or 'the hysterectomy in bed 22'. Sex is a very unwelcome visitor in hospitals; a doctor will often discharge a patient with an A to Z list of dos and don'ts, but there will often not be an 'S' for sexuality on the list.

Research on cancer patients in the 1980s showed that with cancer diagnoses, even though sexual activity decreased, the level of intimacy and need for touch and emotional connectedness became more important.

Our society excludes the disabled and the ill from the fantasy model of sex. To have sex when you have an illness, conditions need to be optimum, and you need to be sexually flexible. Intercourse may not be possible, so you may need to explore 'outercourse'. If you have someone who is ill, and the partner is a carer, there are changes to the dynamics of the relationship, because the carer is more like a parent and the patient is more like a child. So there needs to be a deliberate space made for the sexual relationship to still occur.

For example, once the carer has given attention or medication to the partner there needs to be a physical break from one another. Take a shower, change clothing and meet each other as adult to adult, lover to lover, rather than carer-parent to patient-child. If we wait for sex to happen spontaneously in this situation, often it won't.

When one partner is facing a serious or terminal illness the well partner may try to protect himself or herself from the anticipation of pain and loss by distancing themselves from the sick partner. You may get a situation where one partner needs to be really close, yet the other partner is dealing with his or her grief by creating emotional distance.

When Joy Davidman, the wife of English author C.S. Lewis, was dying of bone cancer she said 'The pain, then, is part of the pleasure now'. What she meant was that if you really love somebody there is always the pain of the risk of losing them. What would you rather do? forgo the love and not have the pain, or experience the love and accept that the pain is simply part of loving someone dearly? David Smarsh, who wrote *The Sexual Crucible*, said, 'It takes tremendous courage to love right up to the moment of death'.

People going through a transition from illness to health need to recognise that there is a grief process necessary in the face of any loss. These losses may be tangible or intangible. The tangible ones are alterations in body image – amputation, hair loss, radiation scarring, surgical scarring, tracheotomy, colonoscopy and the changes in sexual functioning. What may have been possible before may no longer be possible. People need space to grieve those losses.

The intangible ones are loss of the fantasy future. In our own minds we often have a script about how things are going to be, and illness can disrupt this fantasy future. We need to grieve for it even though it is intangible, and then create a new fantasy future. We need to rewrite our life script to incorporate illness or disability in a way that enhances rather than diminishes us.

People who are physically disabled don't fit into normal ideals of what is beautiful, and their sexual development and expression are very much moderated by the attitudes of society and their caretakers. There are rehab programs for all areas of life function, but sex is ignored because disabled people don't fit into this stereotype.

Society has this tendency to assume everyone in a wheelchair is the same, or everyone with a developmental delay is the same, but they are extremely individual with the same differences in potential for sexual expression, joy and sharing. As health-care professionals it is part of holistic patient care that we look after the sexual needs of our patients, as well as their physical, emotional and intellectual needs.

Menopause is a state of hormone deprivation. It affects cognitive functions, which result in problems with memory, concentration and decision-making. This can be extremely distressing. Muscle strength and durability is affected by the drop in testosterone levels, with a resultant muscular fatigue.

Hormone replacement therapy (HRT) can be extremely helpful in reducing the incidence of heart disease, preventing osteoporosis, as well as improving general well-being. When a woman's oestrogen levels drop down her skin sensitivity decreases, her sense of smell decreases, her pheromone amount decreases and this reduces her sense of sexuality. She swaps the scent of a woman for the scent of a grandmother, and going on to HRT can restore these very important functions.

But menopause is not just a hormonal change – it is usually accompanied by many other changes in life. Often it's a change of identity, there is an empty nest or a change in the primary relationship as difficulties become more pronounced. As children leave home the role of being co-parents is lost. There can also be the issue of having older, still dependent children. It's a time when there are changes for men, too, such as retrenchment, depression, alcohol problems or sexual difficulties. Many start taking medication for the first time. And women in our society are not valued as sexual when menopausal. As Joanne Woodward said of her husband Paul Newman, 'He gets prettier and I get older'.

For decades menopausal women have been given oestrogen and progestogen as hormone replacement. While they have had physical and emotional benefits, they haven't had any benefit in the area of sexual desire. When the ovaries stop producing oestrogen and progestogen there is also a reduction in testosterone levels, which has a significant effect on female sex drive. Oestrogen and progestogen have a beneficial effect on sexual response, but not on sexual drive. They actually lower any levels of testosterone remaining in the body so that a woman can find that HRT will be the end of her sex drive. Now we give a woman testosterone replacement as well to help with her sex drive.

For many women menopause is the excuse they have been looking for to give up a sex life that they have never found rewarding. Other women are quite happy to accept the changes and to alter their sexual activity to encompass these and there are some women who say they enjoy sex more. The women who find it more enjoyable no longer have the fear of pregnancy, or an improved personal relationship.

Aging is much more of a challenge for women than it is for men because that is the end of women's reproductive capacity, while men continue their reproductive capacity until they die. In Western society men are valued for what they do and what they have, and as their power and status increase (often with age) they are seen as more sexually attractive. Women are valued by the way they look, so the characteristics that are seen as 'sexy' in a woman such as smooth skin, a slim body and firm breasts, decline much earlier in life than in men.

Our visual media perpetuate these stereotypes, Sean Connery is considered very sexy while Angela Lansbury is a 'granny'. Films increasingly depict older men with increasingly younger women, but you don't see it the other way around. The alternative is plastic surgery, so that women look artificially age-free, for instance Priscilla Presley, Raquel Welch and Jane Fonda. These women are admired for remaining eternally youthful, making aging more and more a taboo for women.

EXERCISE: FINDING YOUR OWN RIGHT CONDITIONS FOR SEX

Given the right conditions arousal is possible. Burnie Zilbergeld, author of Men and Sex, has an exercise where you think of the three best sexual experiences. If you have never had a good sexual experience imagine what one would be like and write down all the reasons why it made that experience good. They could be privacy, having plenty of time, an exciting place, an adventurous sexual activity, a comfortable place, being with someone you love or feeling good about your body.

Next, think about your three worst experiences. If you have never had a bad experience imagine what would be bad for you and write down all the reasons that make it bad. What you have is a list of your positive and negative conditions for sex.

6

Domination and Submission

Surveys of people's sexual fantasies are always fascinating. One of the most interesting aspects of these peeks into the fantasy realm is to see where fantasies differ according to age, gender or sexual preference. Just as fascinating is where these indicators make no difference to the type of fantasies at all. And the number one area where this is the case is domination and submission, where fantasies of being overpowered show up strongly and consistently. It seems that most of us, at least some of the time, fantasise of being dominated and forced into sex. For many this also involves physical discipline of some sort, from having our bottoms playfully spanked, to being severely whipped.

Most people do not act on these fantasies, content to leave them in an imaginary erotic world. For those who do, the results can be profound, with many people reporting that this type of sexual adventure has reignited their relationship's sexual flame. It can reintroduce excitement back into a relationship that has been bogged down in the familiar. To have good SM (sadomasochism) play requires planning, building anticipation and a dramatic flair, and this level of communication and forward planning is great for any couple's sexuality.

Some people go further and decide to permanently incorporate aspects of dominant and submissive roles into not only their sexual expression, but their daily life. These couples take on an SM lifestyle that is not only physically intense, but has an often unexpected spiritual dimension. However, the deep love between an SM couple, which often seems to break all the rules on what makes a good relationship, can be a shock to other people.

For people wanting to get into SM but with no way to access the scene a visit to a professional dominatrix is a great first step. This gives a safe, professional introduction to the scene and a way to learn SM etiquette, how to set limits, discuss fantasies and be introduced to the range of dominant-submissive erotic possibilities. Alternatively if there is a private SM organisation or social club that organises events this would be a good way to learn safety and socialising techniques. It is important to get support because amateurs can often make mistakes.

One of the hardest things SM players have to deal with is the widespread misunderstanding about SM from those outside the scene. People who know nothing of the structure of SM play often view SM as not only non-consensual, but abuse or open to being abused. SM play and activities are always consensual, fully negotiated, with activities agreed to ahead of time. SM players do this to minimise risks to each other's physical and emotional well-being, and to make sure that all parties get what they want from the interaction: erotic pleasure and/or personal growth.

Often people get scared by SM paraphernalia – leather, rubber, studs and whips and chains. For others it is just the outward manifestation of domination and submission that turns them on. Yet while these props and this look can reinforce domination, they do not make a dominant a convincing wielder of power. That comes from within.

Domination and submission play can cover everything from teasingly making someone your sex 'slave' for an hour, to a long, severely painful session of discipline and sexual torture. Bondage and discipline (BD) is the most well-known aspect of SM, but only one part of its rich tapestry. Nevertheless it is the one most people are familiar with and the one that is most subject to nudge-nudge sexual jokes and innuendos. Some definitions:

Top: the dominant partner in dominant-submissive play.

Bottom: the submissive partner in dominant-submissive play.

Switch: refers to someone who can play either dominant or submissive role in sexual play or to a dominant-submissive play session where players change roles halfway through.

Play: doing an SM scene is often called 'playing' because you are actually play-acting out a fantasy role. It is an extension of a childhood game of dress-ups.

Fetish: objects, parts of the body, certain clothes or types of materials can all trigger sexual feelings for people who have a fetish for them. The most well-known material fetishes are fur, leather or rubber. A fetishism for shoes or boots is the most common clothing fetish. A fetish can be mild or extreme, where the material is essential to sexual arousal.

For most people and couples SM begins and ends in their own private space, or in a discreet SM environment. Some women who are involved in the scene in a personal way eventually make a career out of their natural dominant talents and work as professional mistresses. Likewise there are many women who work professionally as mistresses who have no personal interest in SM in their private lives.

In this chapter Cléo Dubois, Kat Sunlove and Amanda Dwyer share decades of experience in the role of erotic domination and submission and their tips on how to recreate this fantasy at home.

KAT SUNLOVE

The desire to be helpless and the wish to yield power

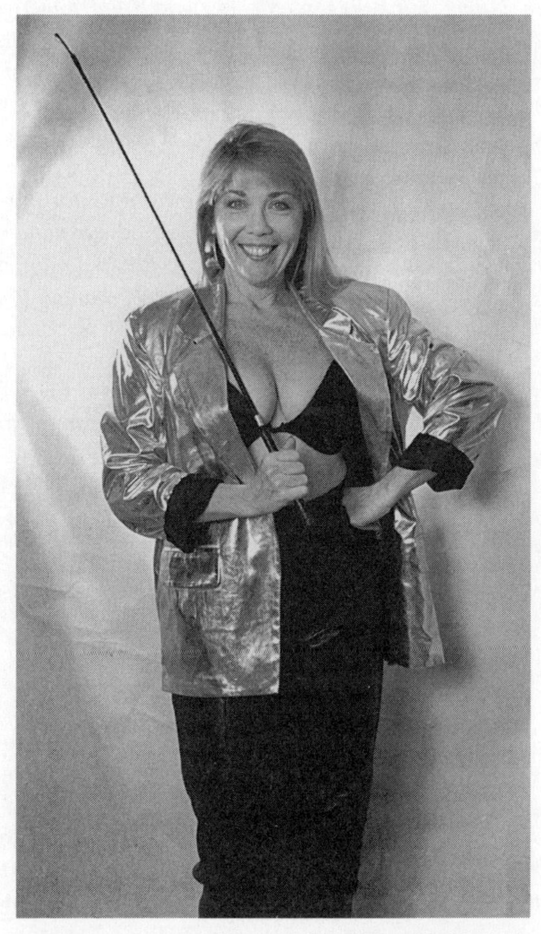

Layne Winklebleck

Since the early 1980s Kat Sunlove has been involved in the sex industry as a performer, journalist, educator, publisher of Spectator and since late 1997, as lobbyist for the Free Speech Coalition. With a Masters in Political Science, a year of law school and many years of political activism, Kat is well-suited for the challenges of advocating for the interests of the sex industry in Sacramento, California and across the US.

Better known as Mistress Kat to her submissive fans, Kat wrote a weekly advice column on erotic dominance and submission for four years in the early 1980s in Spectator and later for the national magazine Chic, earning her the label of the Dear Abby of SM. With her life partner, Layne Winklebleck, she designed and taught a popular workshop series entitled SM for Loving Couples, the first serious educational workshops on this sensational and misunderstood topic. The workshops were featured in an anthropological study of the San Francisco SM community, Erotic Power, *by Dr Gini Graham Scott.*

Kat and Layne have been guest lecturers at San Francisco State University, University of the Pacific and the Institute for the Advanced Study of Human Sexuality. They have appeared on numerous radio and television programs dealing with erotic fantasy play, censorship and sexual freedom. For several years the couple worked to produce a major theatrical production starring Mistress Kat on the theme of erotic female dominance.

Kat was a contributor to the original Cyborgasm CD project, now distributed through Time-Warner and was the inspiration for the first radical sex photo book by Michael Rosen, Sexual Magic: The S/M Photographs. In 1995 Kat produced and starred in her own Fabulous at Fifty Fantasy Ball to celebrate her birthday as well as to promote the idea of the sexiness of older women.

She is a member of Feminists for Free Expression, NOW, COYOTE, the San Francisco Press Club, the Society of Professional Journalists and was a founder of the anticensorship group Cal-ACT. She now serves as the Executive Director of National ACT.

For some years in the early 1980s my life partner, Layne Winklebleck, and I conducted what we've been told were the first-ever serious workshops on erotic dominance and submission or SM. Inspired by our own very self-conscious erotic adventures in this mysterious world of power, we felt that we could help other loving couples pass some of the pitfalls of such an intimate exploration of the darker side of our psyches. It is, after all, a scary place to go: the desire to be helpless, to be taken, to be swept away by another's desire. Or conversely, the wish to inflict pain or wield power over another for one's own selfish sexual gratification. Or so it all appears to the uninitiated. In fact, it's much more complex than that and much more profound.

As Layne and I began playing with power in our own lovemaking, I was struck by the intense erotic thrill I got from his dominant attentions. At this point in my life, age thirty-four, I was identifying as a lesbian, having found men to be too much work. But Layne, a long-time friend, was different. I trusted him and had lusted after him; I knew the quality of his character. So when he put his hand on my throat during sex, I relaxed and enjoyed the delicious sensations that coursed through my body.

Afterwards, I questioned him endlessly, trying to understand what could be so exciting about submitting to a man when I felt that submission to men was largely what had gotten women into the second-class mess we were in. His communication skills and understanding of the human mind, honed by years as a therapist and as a teacher of social work graduate students, enabled him to gently lead me into a deeper and deeper exploration of these amazing energies. Almost in spite of myself, I was drawn into this taboo world of power play. The experiences were telepathic. We would each feel a dark thrill – a growling, blood-thickening rush, we called it – when our respective mental and emotional states were tuned into each other like some errant radio wave that finally finds the right channel. He, the lustful, harsh master; I, the willing, accepting slave.

And still, as much as I came to enjoy and appreciate my submissive side, I could not fathom wanting to hurt him or to dominate him. But I was curious. He suggested that I try slapping him during a lovemaking session one night when I was atop him. I gave his face a light blow, and we laughed at my reticence. Then he said, 'Go ahead, try again. I'll still love you even if you hurt me.' Unable to resist the challenge, I let go and slapped full-out. The rush I felt was frightening to me, so strongly did it throb in my cunt. By pushing past my own limits, I had discovered my sadistic potential. But I was afraid of it, fearful that I would actually hurt someone in order to feel that thrill.

By continuing our explorations, both together and with others, however, I learned that I would not hurt anyone. I merely seek out those who would enjoy and revel in the other side of that erotic dyad. We also learned that there are some emotional risks in this kind of play. You must know and trust your partner. And your partner must be trustworthy. Safe words don't matter to a psychopath, so you have to be sure that the person you choose to play with is sane. The submissive must be able ultimately to take care of their own needs, to ask for love and gentleness when the dominant forgets to show affection. The dominant must always remember it's a game intended for pleasure and they must not slip over the edge from pushing limits to violating them.

Eventually, I turned the tables on Layne and became the dominant of his dreams and he, the submissive of dreams I never really knew I had. We threw ourselves into a pursuit of knowledge and experience of this misunderstood area of human sexuality. For almost a year, we read everything we could find on the subject (not much) and experimented with lifestyle dominance and submission, but eventually found that it was not for us.

We decided that the oppression both sexes feel in modern society is role-based, not gender-based. In other words, the dominant, whether male or female, gets tired of always making the decisions, initiating the action, taking care of the bottom. Similarly, the submissive may begin to feel unappreciated, under-loved or misused by the top. Both can feel taken for granted if there is not enough 'straight time', time to be real and talk about one's feelings, about what is working for each and what is not. Communication in this arena, just as in many other parts of life, is the key. People who are not honest with themselves or who do not know themselves well and who do not listen to their partner are often unable to achieve the personal growth and erotic satisfaction available through SM play. They can get lost in their own fantasies and mistake submission for stupidity, dominance for callousness.

In our workshops, we focused on female dominance and male submission, not because of an erotic bias, but rather because that had been the direction of our greatest learning and because we felt that was the direction most likely to benefit society. To help a man get in touch with his desire for submission, to allow a woman room to explore her dominant fantasies, seemed likely to help both. To get a woman in touch with her own erotic power and to use that power lovingly with a partner, to help her understand why he wants and needs the experience of submission – these were the motivations we had in designing our workshops.

Our messages were simple. To the women we said, 'Find your own dominant style, explore your own fantasies. Listen to his fantasies but only as fuel for your own. Use what you like and stay true to your own energy. Plan ahead. Tease, tease, tease. Create a fantasy world of your own in which you can have your sexual desires fulfilled. Play safe. Try the equipment on yourself so you know what you are doing to his body. A crop hurts far more than a flogger, despite their relative appearance. Stay sane. Go far enough to 'scratch his itch' but not so far as to really do harm. Hypnotise him with voice, eyes, touch. Tune into him and follow the energy. Show him your love and your magnificence as well as your dominance.'To the men we said, 'Let go of your fantasised wants and let her use you for her desires. Be genuine in your submission. Love her dominant self. Respect her. Let yourself be taken. Be patient as she learns the ropes. Never leave egg on her face by telling her she isn't doing it right. Don't be so goal-orientated. Enjoy the flow of energy. Open up and let her see your soft side. Relax, relax and breathe.'We didn't encourage so-called safe words. Instead, we put the dominant in charge and made her fully responsible for staying in control of safety as well as sex. We did encourage straight time for communicating outside of the bedroom or dungeon.

One of the most important lessons we tried to teach the men was how to introduce the idea of SM play to their female partner. Having indulged in only isolated masturbatory fantasies of submission, many men may start with some extreme image that has evolved over many years. My advice was not to begin, for instance, with a castration fantasy. That would probably turn her off. Start with something simple and non-threatening, spanking perhaps, or gentle scarf bondage. He should ask her what her fantasies are instead of focusing only on his own. Many women, for example, have dreamed of a love slave who would service them sexually, but have not put that fantasy into a power context. Introduce the idea of being that love slave by offering a massage or a foot rub, followed by lengthy oral sex if she enjoys that.

Most of all, we say to both parties, stay true to oneself. If the energy is not there, stop. Talk. Try something else. Try again another time. Laugh. Be playful with one another and forgiving of the mis-steps. Remember that it's a mysterious world we enter when we try to actualise erotic fantasy. But it's also a magical sharing of intimate parts of ourselves that can bring us closer together. When it works, it's wonderful.

TIPS FOR WOMEN WANTING TO EXPLORE DOMINANCE

• Start with an attitude. Be playful, adventuresome, curious about what you'll learn. Be willing to explore your sexuality, your capacity for sadism. Build your self-confidence with clothing, toys, treats. Love his submission; appreciate your dominance. Maintain your integrity – do it for yourself.

• Trust the energy. Trust the mutuality of the energy – if you're hot, he's hot. Open up the intimate parts of yourself – desire to know his intimate parts as well and don't judge him badly when he shares them. Look at your dark sides and determine to explore them together – the yin and yang.

• Get yourself turned on first – horny is good! Put yourself in action mode – no lazy dominants. Feel sexy, use your body and hands to tease. Fantasise, fantasise! Find archetypes to emulate: goddess image, powerful women, mothers.

• Create an illusion. Be a `method' actress and find the energy from within. Read his energy and manipulate it. Look into his eyes, watch his cock, check his breathing for clues to his arousal. Plan ahead. Set things up beforehand – surprise him with a new toy, then use it on him.

• Let go of guilt – these energies are natural and positive. See yourself as an object of his desire, that he wants you! Know that it is a mutually pleasurable experience. Know that only you can give him what he needs. If you're angry at him, don't play – SM is not real punishment.

• Find the edge, the rush, and follow that energy. Remember him at some level, for safety's sake. Make it real by doing more than he expects, more than you expect. Start where you are comfortable – scratching, light bondage, spanking.

• Create sensation in his body and in yours – pleasure is okay too. Strip him of control – you take control – forbid a hard-on! Tie it behind him. Use body language, facial expressions. Toys are everywhere, in the kitchen, bath, bedroom, fingernails, hair, anything that can create sensation at your command.

• Hypnotise him. Tell him how you want him to be; teach him. Use your voice, making it soft, stern, rhythmically paced. Touch softly, seduce him. Help him relax (very important!). 'Spacing out' is profound submission – let him.

• Find out what he likes, what his fantasies are. Have him keep a journal, send you cards with his private thoughts. Decide which of his fantasies you like and use them on him. Give him a ride – the thrill of the roller-coaster, a loss of control. Talk to him about what you're going to do to him and see how he reacts. If there's no charge there, you don't have to follow through.

• Beware of the problems: feeling like his 'whore' because you are doing it for him; feeling responsible for his experience and therefore feeling inadequate if it doesn't work; the pressure to be creative (when in doubt, blindfold him); the elusive erection (just because he doesn't get hard doesn't mean he's not excited). Make sure you have 'straight' time to be real with each other and talk about the experience.

CLÉO DUBOIS

The journey to dark Eros

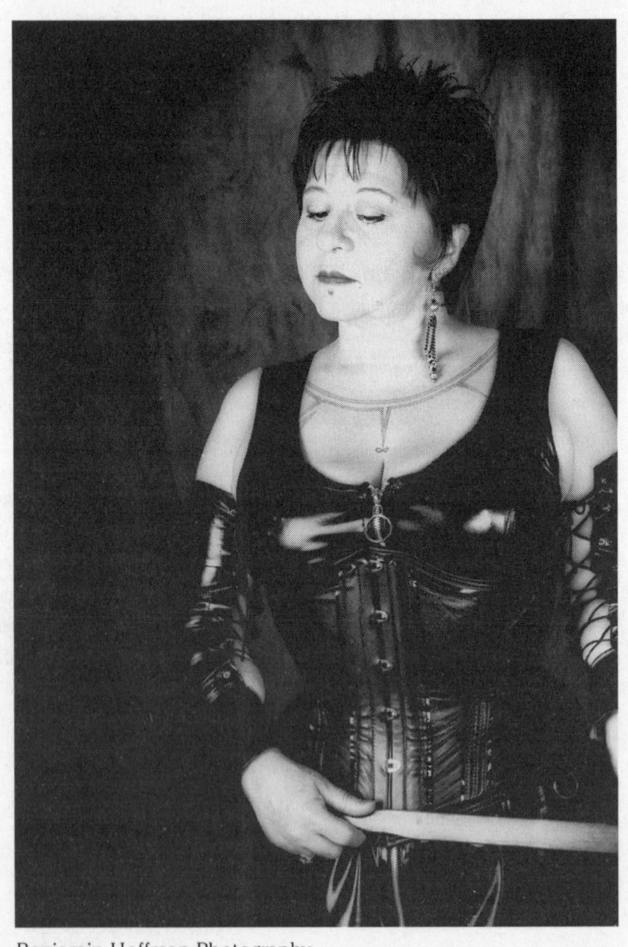

Benjamin Hoffman Photography

Born and raised in Paris, France, in the early 1980s Cléo Dubois began exploring the SM frontiers in the San Francisco leather community. After attending her first, then very underground, workshop given by Mistress Kat and Layne, she devoted herself to learning BD (bondage and discipline) and SM skills and safety, both as a top and a bottom. Within a year, she became an enthusiastic, responsible, caring sadist.

Today, with her Academy of SM Arts, Cléo is a highly respected BD/SM educator and Domina, as well as an active member of the San Francisco leather community, and private player. Cleo is a sought-after speaker for such established organisations as Differences, QSM, Society of Janus, and NLA Living in Leather conferences, and APEX in Arizona. She is profiled in the book Different Loving.

An in-depth interview with her by Carol Queen appeared in the 1998 Bitch Goddess, edited by Pat Califia and Drew Campbell. She has been featured in Boudoir Noir, Skin Two, Prometheus *and* Sexual Magic *by Michael A. Rosen. As an educator and body ritual performer she has appeared at London's ICA, and Festival Atlantico in Lisbon, Portugal, and was featured on French television as part of 'Canal +' series on alternative cultures.*

Coming out into her sadism and masochism was a powerful and liberating experience for me. I was born and raised in France, where erotic SM has been part of an underground élite culture for centuries. I think, perhaps, that made it easier for me to be proud of my dominant sadism.

As a child, however, I was bullied, dominated, tormented and humiliated by my male cousins. Power was used by my father over me, my mother and my peers in an abusive manner. I learned early to distrust and question that sort of authority and to rebel and fight back. As a result I developed inner strength and great independence.

I travelled alone a lot in my early twenties and was outraged at the many ways women were controlled by males in societies governed by patriarchal religions, especially in the Middle East. Whether it was their brothers, fathers or husbands women didn't have the right to own their bodies, their sexuality or even their own pleasure! At that time, personally I manipulated men through the usual tease and denial tactics learned in my Catholic upbringing.

In 1981, in San Francisco, I attended an SM workshop and immediately found the link to my sexuality that was missing. My sadism came into focus. Playing with power consensually and erotically made all the difference – this was no longer abuse! In my work today, I help couples and singles with the many skills it takes to safely explore loving bondage and SM role-play. I see this as a way to increase intimacy between players and create what I call 'sensual magic' and 'the journeys to dark Eros'. My expertise and sensitivity enable me to share the secret of successful kinky play stressing trust, negotiation, turn-on, technical skills, risks and rewards and the passionate excitement of it all. Since all BD/SM interaction involves negotiation, I first reassure those who contact me that everything they say will remain confidential. A basic lesson I've learned is just how difficult it is for many of us to communicate our erotic needs.

I've learned to ask many questions, the most important of these being `What do you mean by that?'. I ask what psychological and physical elements are in the person's fantasy. 'Who are you in the fantasy?' `Are you a willing submissive?' 'A masochist who wants to explore limits?' 'A play slave?' 'A servant?' 'A captive?' 'What sort of activity takes place?' 'Are there any recurring trigger words or images that turn you on?' I do not attempt to act out scripted fantasies because when people create their fantasies, they are in control of all the elements. When they communicate a fantasy to others, they cannot stay in full control. The acted-out fantasy will never match up to the idea they keep in their heads. I will never be able to take them anywhere real in this kind of situation. Therefore the drama that unfolds must be genuinely collaborative. If I'm only an actress, I don't get a sense of my own power and my intuition is stifled. Having creativity allows me to be powerful and intuitive, and keeps the dynamic exciting and hot.

In terms of my own sexuality playing with an enormous range of people of all ages and from all walks of life has taught me to never say 'never'. It has taught me how rich and diverse are the ways that people express their sexuality. Ten years ago, for example, I had little or no understanding of men who sought to explore their female personae, and even thought that cross-dressing degraded women. Now I appreciate gender role reversal, especially if the situation is kinky and involves a helpless slut or French maid! I've also learned to be aware of the necessity of honouring my own needs as a 'switch' in my private life. Being on the dominant side too much can push me off-balance: I know that bottoming in my private life will psychically and erotically recharge me. Unfortunately I do not have as much desire as I would like to top my lovers if they, too, need to be tied up, teased, tormented and thoroughly done! Another thing that has happened is I've discovered my bisexuality – I cherish the expression of my kinkiness with women as well as with men.

The single most important thing I do to separate the professional SM mistress from my intimate relationship, which I've done from the beginning, is to treat the dungeon as a sacred space, a temple, a sanctuary. What happens in the dungeon happens in a different space, in a different, magical, time. It bears no relation to the rest of my life. In addition to this, I maintain certain boundaries with my clients. Like a therapist, I do not socialise with them. I keep my personal and professional lives very separate. I do not work five days a week. I do not, under any circumstances, 'bottom' professionally, I need to keep that space for my private life.

Many people ask how they can get a stranger, or someone new, to open up about their fantasies and live them out in an SM scene. People want to know how to set up boundaries beforehand to make it safe for those involved. If you find yourself in a situation where you are going on a kinky path for the first time with a lover, or perhaps someone you know less well, you need to communicate your fantasies, your expertise and your experience. What do you want? How compatible are you? How experienced are you? These aren't necessarily easy questions. The SM scene isn't something ready-made that you then act out together. It depends on both parties being able to identify their desires, and to courageously and honestly start expressing them. What do you really want? What does your lover really want? You might not be willing to reveal all the dark, sticky, scary, weird stuff your fantasies are made of. What are you willing to reveal, to explore with this other person? Be clear and brave about what you want and what you are willing to do.

This honesty comes with a risk: your lover might say no, be horrified or put off – the risk of rejection. Remember that you have the right to fantasise about whatever you want – fantasy alone never hurt anyone. Being rejected, however, does hurt, so know that that's a possibility. You need to decide who wants to do what to whom. From my long experience with working with couples, I know that it is surprisingly common for lovers to both be switches, or even bottoms. How to negotiate this? Parity, making sure that everyone's needs or desires are met at least some of the time, can mean taking turns. Even though SM people are usually not swingers, but players, they can seek out, with the consent of their partners, other part-time play-partners outside the relationship with whom they can play different games. In most cases, once we've started to really explore our erotic BD/SM desires, it really isn't viable to keep our activities to just one partner.

Now, let's suppose your lover wants to be tied up, but you don't know the first thing about knots. Let's also suppose he or she wants to be spanked for being naughty, and then shamelessly made love to. You might enjoy the idea of making your lover into a slave for the evening, to serve you dessert with a collar around the neck wearing nothing but a lacy apron and high-heeled shoes.

In the negotiation, find out about any physical limitations your partner may have, such as bad knees or a bad back. Ask about phobias and fears, trigger words that could be hurtful, as well as what they really crave. Give your bottom a safe word. Everyone in California is very familiar with 'yellow' for 'please slow down, caution, I'm almost at my limit, I need a break' and 'red' for stop. For the bottom to implore 'Please, please stop' is often a turn-on and can be part of the scene, so the safe word is important to distinguish between fantasy and reality. If you both agree that this could be fun, then this is how to start to play.

EXERCISE: YOUR FIRST SM SCENE WITH SOMEONE NEW

First, set up a special evening for your scene. You'll need a good three or four hours for the whole scene. Instruct your partner on what to wear and what to bring with them. Ask them to find and buy a frilly apron and some sexy high-heeled shoes. Have your equipment ready too.

For this scene, you'll need candles, a dog collar that fits your bottom's neck, with a chain – these can be found at the supermarket as well as in a leather store – maybe some light bondage wrist-cuffs. A sleep-mask or a blindfold. A piece of nylon rope, not longer than 3 metres, and not too thin – twine can cut. Look around the kitchen and see what catches your eye. A wooden kitchen spoon makes a great spanking implement, as does a small wooden chopping board, or a wooden back-scratcher if you have one.

Find some clothes pegs to use as nipple clamps. Have fun thinking of erotic uses for everyday household objects! Unplug the phone. Set the scene with some low lighting, maybe some candles, and some sensuous or evocative music. If you want a more Victorian feel, play some Mozart! Pick your costume carefully (you might, at some point, order your slave to undress you and fold your clothes neatly, while on their hands and knees).

Take a comfortable seat, take a few deep breaths, be centred, and call in your slave. Tell him or her to come close to you and be seen. Have him or her slowly undress before you and fold their clothes in a neat pile on the floor. On their hands and knees, have them put the clothes to one side while you watch them crawl. Comment on their form, on their beauty, like you would a fine new acquisition. Caress your new toy gently and slowly.

Order him or her to kneel before you. Take the collar in your hands. Stand up and ask if he or she is ready to accept your collar as a symbol of willing submission. Say how you wish to be addressed: Sir, Madam, My Lady, Lord, Master or Mistress. Ask him or her to tell you what the safe words are, to ensure everyone remembers. Take control of your slave's actions. Do you want his or her eyes lowered to the floor, or looking up at you? Keep your orders simple and precise. See how they are followed. Be just: if your slave is good and attentive, he or she should be rewarded, touched sweetly, turned-on.

If the service is bad, if your drink is spilled, give your slave five good whacks with the wooden spoon. It is possible that your partner might be sassy and even seek some light humiliation or more pain. How does that feel? Don't get angry, remember you are both playing. It's only by experimenting with acting out your fantasy that you will discover who your play persona is – master, trainer, interrogator, brat, good girl/boy, smart-arsed masochist or true submissive slave.

Play, and have fun. You might want to place the clothes pegs on your slave's nipples, just to see how he or she responds to a little pain. Make sure you look into your partner's eyes when you remove them after a few minutes, and take notice of your own reaction – could you have a sadistic streak? You might want to use the rope to tie your submissive's hands behind his or her back or to a chair, or cuff and tie him or her to the bed. Simple knots are always the best, and make sure to have a pair of scissors handy just in case.

Blindfolding your bound lover and tormenting him or her with gentle sensual touching will heighten the perception of your touch. Playing with trust and surrender in this way can be a fabulous turn-on. Your hands, your voice, your mouth, your breath are also your toys, so use them to full effect. Your power doesn't come from the rope or wooden spoon, but from you. All these things are but extensions of your power and energy, emanating from your core. Be centred, feel your power, feel the turn-on that you create for yourself and your partner.

Be open to the exchange of energy between the two of you. Try shifting the power around?get really close to your bottom, whisper softly, touch sweetly, breathe warm breath on your lover's neck. Stand apart, take charge with your voice, run your nails across his or her skin. Use contrasts in sensations. Your hands can touch sweetly, but can also rub, pinch and scratch. Don't ask for permission. Pay attention to the responses, your partner's breathing and level of turn-on.

Don't be shy to ask for what you really want your bottom specifically to do for you. Maybe you want your breasts touched and kissed in a certain way. Perhaps you wish your lover to worship your feet and ankles. Tell him or her exactly how you like it, how you want it done. Guide your partner so he or she can serve you in the best possible way. Be present for the turn-on that brings. Use breathing techniques to keep centred: deep breathing increases awareness of our being in our bodies, and makes it easier to project our power outward. In this way you create a ritualised, magical scene. I strongly believe in the magic of SM and intimacy games.

Find your power. Feel it, use it, play with it, and above all, enjoy it. This scene might not have much heavy SM or bondage, and maybe it will lead to some great, hot straight sex, but that's just the point. You've opened the door, got a taste, and the future is wide open. Remember, you collared your partner as a symbol of your dominance and his or her submission. It is your responsibility to remove it, and to close the scene when the play is ended. Talking about the scene the next day, or within a few days, is also very important.

Exploring our fantasy lives can raise questions of what is consensual power play and what is real abuse. The SM credo, as is well-known, is that play must be safe, sane and consensual. Nonetheless, many things can happen in the context of a scene when limits are reached and challenged. Emotional damage often cannot be anticipated. A certain judgement made in a scene might cut like a knife to the heart; our fears over our inadequacies might be powerfully and painfully triggered – our high can turn into a painful dive into depression and fear of rejection. This can be equally true from a top or a bottom perspective.

In terms of physical damage, what's important is to be educated about what is and isn't safe to play with. At the end of the twentieth century there is a great deal of concrete information out there, both in non-fiction books and on the World Wide Web.

AMANDA DWYER

Nothing to fear

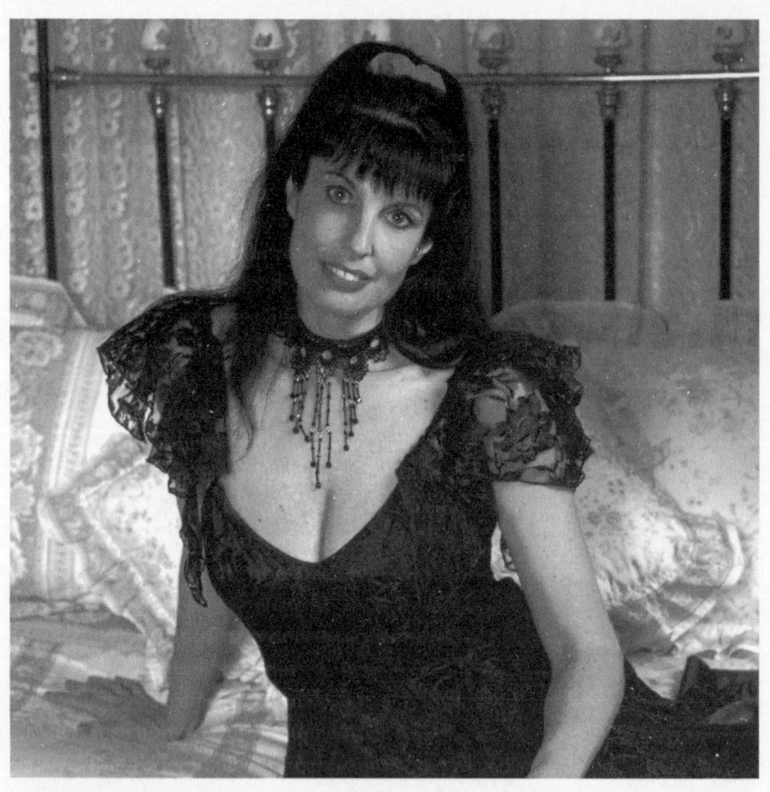

Amanda Dwyer began her career as a mistress in 1986 with an apprenticeship at Salon Kitty's, which had been established four months earlier as a brothel. It soon began specialising in BD and fantasy services, with a core of experienced mistresses from around Sydney.

Amanda's natural flair and attraction to SM, plus her sense of organisation and former business experience soon resulted in her coming to the notice of Salon Kitty's owner. What was intended to be a dalliance with the scene saw her being given a management position within the establishment. In 1989, she bought the business outright.

Like most people who are into the SM scene, dominance and submission had been part of Amanda's psyche from an early age. Like many people, she was unable to recognise this until she saw an advertisement for apprentice mistresses. She responded and spending one day among the extraordinary women who are mistresses and submissives in a professional establishment was enough to convince her.

Amanda has advocated for the BD and SM scene and the sex industry in general. In 1990, Amanda was part of a movement aimed at legalising and legitimising the sex industry in New South Wales and for a year was the industry's main spokesperson.

Amanda has often been called the 'Queen of BDSM in Australia', but still continues to conduct sessions at Salon Kitty's. After thirteen years in the profession, one-to-one sessions remain the most important expression of her SM life. She says 'it has become my business, but most importantly, it is a fundamental part of my personality'.

I have appeared repeatedly in the media in an educational role, not to evangelise BD and SM, but to demystify it. I believe that it is a form of expression important to only a minority of people, but to those people it is a crucial part of their life. I have always sought to demonstrate that there is nothing to fear from BD or SM. As long as the basic tenets of 'safe, sane and consensual' are followed, then BD and SM are just expressions of human sexuality and interaction.

I don't think my work has been good for my own sexuality. I think I have become so centred on being obliged to constantly give pleasure to others that in my own private life I tend to get a bit `over it all'. My life revolves around hearing and reading, supplying and satisfying men's sexual fantasies. I think it is easy to become a little jaded. I think a lot of what I have experienced over the years makes me realise there are and always will be many differences between men and women on matters of sexual feelings and interest. I know I haven't found all the answers to what gives me a sexual high.

At this point in my life I feel as though I have totally lost touch with my sexuality. I know a lot of women say they don't really know or understand themselves sexually until they reach the age of thirty-five, but I can't say the same goes for me. It isn't that I haven't grown or learned anything over the years, but I do blame my work for interfering with my personal sexual expression. I think by constantly having to satisfy in a commercial sense (no matter what role you may be taking), you have to deliver and there is always something expected from you.

These expectations (put upon myself) tend to invade my personal life. I think I have become afraid of finding my real sexual self. I wouldn't say working in the sex industry has done a great deal for my personal confidence. I think you need to have a certain amount of confidence to feel, and actually be, sexy. Contrary to popular belief, not all who work in the BD/SM scene have the confidence many people assume we possess.

I don't believe women are the superior sex or any woman is a goddess. I do believe women should have equal rights and opportunities just like men. We are an equal part of the human race and still strive to be recognised in many societies today. Some attitudes will take several generations to change.

TIPS: SAFELY EXPLORING BD/SM WITHIN YOUR RELATIONSHIP

• First of all it is necessary that both parties are interested and wanting to be involved. The words 'safe, sane and consensual' are paramount. You must be able to trust your partner – without trust this style of relationship should not be entered into.

• Most people like to take either the dominant or submissive role. I believe it is a good idea when first starting out to try taking on both roles in turns. Most of us have a natural tendency to be dominant or submissive but it never hurts to know just how it feels both physically and emotionally to be in either position.

• It is always important to start off by taking things slowly. It is also a good idea not to try too many activities in the one session as it could be a little overwhelming. BD and SM is a very sexual experience, but it is arousal of a type which you have probably never experienced previously.

• Try sensory deprivation. It is amazing how the body feels when you are lightly restrained and unable to hear or see. Physical sensations seem to increase dramatically.

• Many people find it difficult to actually put their feelings or desires into words for fear of rejection or disapproval. It is paramount that people inform partners of levels of interest and experience, and obey and respect each other's limits.

• Purchase a few basic items from your local sex shop. Wrist and/or ankle restraints, a slave collar that signifies the submissive position, a blindfold for sensory deprivation (this can heighten sexual awareness), some sash cord for basic bondage, long shoe-lacing for genital bondage, a small leather paddle and a riding crop. Clothes pegs can be substituted for nipple clamps (which can be quite expensive). These items are very basic but won't break the budget.

• If you find you like exploring these roles you can purchase other pieces of equipment and discipline implements. Some creative individuals get a lot of fun from making their own toys and equipment. If you fall into this category all the better; hand made pieces are far more personal.

• Finally, once you feel confident in your chosen role you may like to venture a little further by attending BD or SM functions where you can meet up with like-minded people who share your interests. These gatherings can be lots of fun and a good way to make new friends.

7

Female Ejaculation and Oral Sex

Traditionally sex workers have been viewed as victims – women who have had tragic childhoods, are generally unloved, or victims of an unscrupulous man or a serious drug habit. There has been little acceptance that a woman could choose sex work as a short-term or long-term career option and make a success of it. More shocking is the view that women could enjoy sex work or be prostitutes or dominatrixes as well as loving wives and caring mothers.

For some women working in the sex industry has been a negative experience they regret; for others their time in the industry has been a way to learn about human sexuality. Sex workers get a unique look at people's fantasies, insecurities, vulnerabilities and fears. They are front-line sexual researchers and have an untapped body of knowledge that should be respected and documented. Most of them would not give up their sex-industry experiences – either good and bad – for the world.

Many women who have never worked in the sex industry are nonetheless fascinated by the world's oldest profession. For women to watch a strip show or a live erotic performance is to see another woman wield her sexual power in a way that can be erotic and seductive. For many women the sexual fantasy of being a prostitute, from a high-class whore to a sassy street-walker, is a way of playing with being wanted and desired. When a woman fantasises about being a leather-clad dominatrix with her own dungeon of gorgeous slaves she can have an experience of absolute power and control.

To be both a feminist and a sex worker is even more controversial, to feminists and non-feminists alike. It is the feminist sex workers who have offered some of the most important new insights into the sex industry. Unfortunately they have also been the women most attacked by other women as betraying the feminist cause, because they see no contradiction between wanting to overthrow male power and running a sexual service for men.

Many sex workers have to live with the stigma still attached to sex work, meaning they often are forced to run a double life. The stress of having to cover up what you do for a living, and the fear of being found out, can cause extreme personal pressure for individual sex workers. It is important that movements for sexual liberation include rights for sex workers to empowerment and legalisation or decriminalisation of the industry.

Every sex worker knows about oral sex, a standard stock-in-trade for the professional. It is the number one fantasy of most men, and the ability of sex workers to fulfil this dream is highly prized.

Sexuality pioneer Deborah Sundahl demystified the G-spot orgasm and female ejaculation through her best-selling video *How to Female Ejaculate*. In the video her clear explanations and cheeky how-to sessions gave a new, clear insight into this previously little understood phenomenon. Sexually fulfilling a woman by stimulating her G-spot is something every lover of women should know and every woman should experience. Her video and work in this area is the kind of public sexuality education we need.

In this chapter the women who know offer guidance: Deborah Sundahl shares her extraordinary journey from stripper to spiritual sensualist; Dolores French gives a professional's view on oral sex and some expert tips.

DEBORAH SUNDAHL

Spiritual access

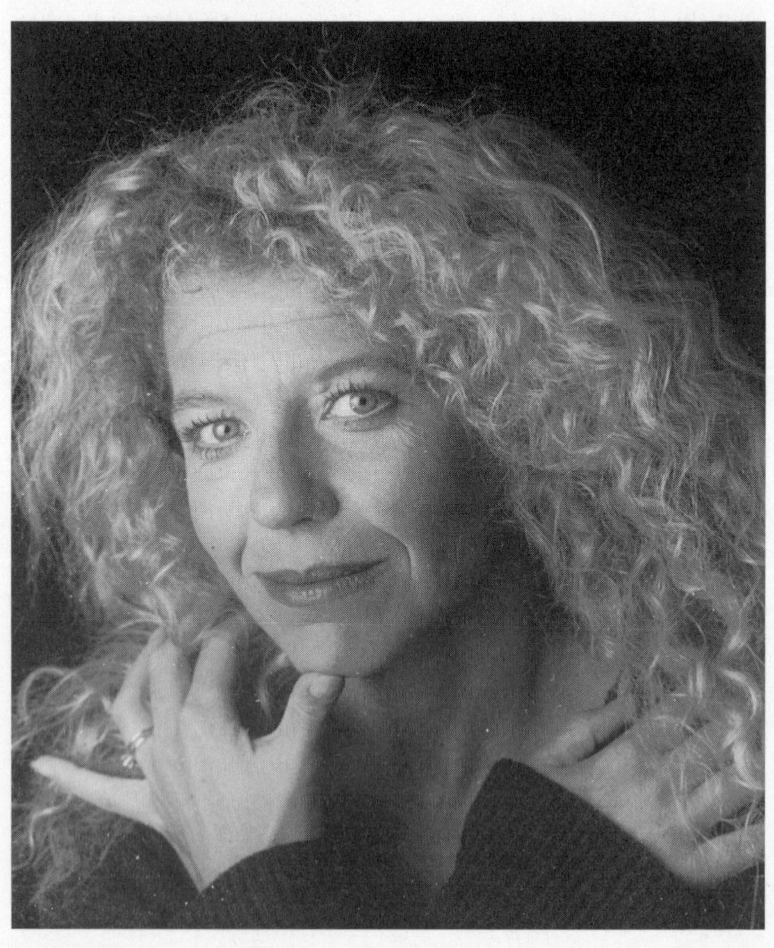

American-born Deborah Sundahl was one of the founders of On Our Backs*, a lesbian erotic magazine that ran for ten years, from 1984 to 1994. It was the mouthpiece for emerging women's erotica - women speaking their sexual desires from their own voice. Many women credit the magazine for changing their lives, and it was the inspiration for many other women's erotic magazines.*

She was also well-known as San Francisco stripper extraordinaire Fanny Fatale, who had her own loyal following. She pioneered the women-only strip shows, Burlezk, and brought the art of striptease to a female-only audience.

She is currently producer of women's educational sex videos, which she calls 'erotica with intelligence and spirit from a woman's point of view'. She specialises in educating about Tantric sex and female ejaculation.

On Our Backs was the first magazine to address sexuality positively and from a woman's point of view. All other magazines at that time were created by men for men's enjoyment. *On Our Backs* addressed important sexual issues for women, such as broadening the definition of the female body, enjoying sex toys, allowing and expressing one's fantasies, exploring gender bending (role reversals) and dominant-submissive play.

The point with *On Our Backs* was to have fun with sex, educate ourselves about the variety of sexual expressions possible in order to foster tolerance, and shed the personal guilt that kept us from our true sexual desires. As a lesbian magazine, *On Our Backs* flew in the face of the conservative, anti-sex lesbian culture that existed at that time, and which mimicked the larger culture's conservative swing. It was liberating, lively and broke sexual taboos continuously in its initial years.

By the time I sold the magazine in 1994, *On Our Backs* had created real cultural change. Sexuality was recognised as the defining force that broadened and unified a newly emerging culture, which included not just lesbians, but gay men, bisexuals and hip, heterosexual couples. They labelled it 'queer'. *On Our Backs*' ideas also began to seep into a stagnant, male-dominated adult industry. Women, both gay and straight, were beginning to have influence for the first time as consumers over what was made and purchased, and they demanded quality.

It was out of this context of destroying old, damaging

stereotypes of female sexuality and birthing new definitions of ourselves from our truth that I suddenly hit a huge wall in my own sexuality. After I left On Our Backs my libido bit the dust, which meant I had nothing more to say or to create with. I had been on the forefront of female sexuality, and now I began to question all I had taught and publicised for ten years. I felt like I was disintegrating, my identity being stripped from me. It was incredibly terrifying, and I felt as raw as someone without skin. I sought out the solace and protection of the deserts of the south-west US to go through this change and sort things out.

The south-west is a very spiritual place, rich in Native American culture, and not very populated. There I could reflect in solitude and anonymity. It became clear that what had started out as a labour of love and intense creativity had turned into a soul-draining management headache. I was juggling a publication deadline, horrendous cashflow endemic to small, counter-culture projects, and the video production and mail-order parts of the business. We tried to grow it, using every tenacious skill we had, but failed. It was a difficult time, and I sold the magazine. I had given all I had and enough was enough. Sitting under a star-filled night, a refugee from the city culture, I began the slow process of diving deep and surfacing with real parts of my lost self.

What began to emerge was a passion for nature and learning to be responsible for my own survival. I began a research trip visiting and working on permaculture and herb farms, and assisting with the building of alternative structures. I learned I had far greater capability to care for myself than our medical establishment and economic structure would like us to believe. When I first stepped into a house made completely of organic material from the earth, heated and powered by the sun, watered by the rains and cleaned by the plants, the nurturing feeling was so overwhelming that I sat down and sobbed.

Meanwhile, my libido had degenerated to the point where I could not touch myself sexually without feeling terribly devastated or lethargic. I knew something new was emerging, requiring me to reject all my well-worn, playful and joyful, nasty and lusty ways. I followed an impulse to practise yoga daily, and this led to an exploration of 'devotional love'. In devotional yoga, one meditates on the subtle feelings, both emotional and physical, that arise in the body while in a yoga position.

One day, to my great surprise, my libido leaped into a raging fire as I sat immersed in contemplation of uniting myself with the cosmic force. So, I meditated on these sexual feelings as I did all the other feelings that arose in my body. I experimented with 'holding' as much erotic pleasure as possible, and with forgoing the urge, almost instinctive in most of us, to immediately satisfy it. There was a period when I did this for hours at a time - when I moved to Santa Fe, New Mexico. I found a place on the edge of a forest where I could meditate in silence and lived like a hermit for two years. The forest, ancient growth in particular, is where my power as a woman lies, and it is fuelled by my sexuality. My spirit is powered and directed by my erotic energy.

Getting in touch with my sexual desires and emotions and giving them voice all those years has obviously led me to desiring to feel the voice of the earth and the whispers of the forest. To express my sexuality and love for another in that context is awesome and exciting, and feels like a vast frontier. I have had to be unpartnered all this time in order to peel away the old sexuality and birth the new Self. I look forward to sharing this greater capacity to express my sexuality in a spiritual context with a new partner someday soon.

After many years of painstaking inner searching, I was able to leave my hermitage. I found I had gained new purpose, and renewed strength and recharged vitality to take with me back out into the work world again. The message I gained was clear: uncovering our sexual fantasies, becoming 'erotically literate' about ourselves, and gaining confidence to communicate our sexual needs successfully, leads to uncovering the real power of our erotic being: spiritual access. This is self-knowledge of a very deep kind. At its core, sexual expression is about learning how to love ourselves and others.

I used to laugh at this concept of love in the early stages of On Our Backs, thinking it too gooey and stereotypical of what a woman was expected to be. At On Our Backs, we felt it was essential that women loosened up sexually and behaved more aggressively. For instance, bend that guy over and drop his pants and do a quickie with a dildo and harness. This sojourn into an all-stops-pulled sexual exploration led me, full circle, back to love. It required a more sobering look at what that feels like in my body, and what that kind of intimacy with another actually requires.

Recently Gina Odgen, a colleague and author of the book Women

Who Love Sex, pointed out that perhaps I had been doing this more intimate, spiritually based loving all along, but simply had not the words to describe or define it as such. I realised that the tenderness and intimacy I felt when embraced in an SM scene was profound. Can one really understand surrender if one has never had one's hands and feet bound and lain helpless in complete trust of the one they love? I have used those experiences to practise surrendering into the tenderness and bliss of someone loving me or myself loving me.

Back in the work world, I considered doing a heterosexual couples' version of my best-selling video *How to Female Ejaculate*, knowing it would sell well and get me back on my feet, but my artistic self refused. Instead, *Journey to Female Orgasm: Awakening the G-spot and Female Ejaculation* was born. I felt it necessary to record this incredible process of transformation, and to help women take those first few steps toward accessing this world of spiritual-sexual power. This video demonstrates how the G-spot is not a magic button for instant gratification, but is instead the opposite: a source of intense physical sensation, deep emotions, and a gateway to accessing consciousness.

This is important news about the G-spot and in the video *Journey to Female Orgasm* I explain how a G-spot massage can heal these old traumatic wounds to our sexual seat, and how it can re-awaken it to its true and powerful potential. When I did *How to Female Ejaculate* in 1991, I feared I'd be run out of town on a rail by saying all woman can ejaculate, because it was so utterly silenced that few people knew about it. Those women who did ejaculate mistook it for peeing in bed and suffered awful embarrassment and shame. Sometimes their husbands left them, or they simply stopped without even being aware that they had the capability to control ejaculation.

Ejaculation, in women and men, can be controlled. Women have learned to control it almost completely and men have learned to control it hardly at all. This is a huge imbalance between the sexes sexually that Tantric practices have done much to correct.

Today, female ejaculation is more understood and even popularised, and so I want to take it to the next level. This level parallels my sexual process from political liberation to spiritual awakening. A new century is upon us that demands we live on this earth and treat ourselves and others on a much higher, loving level than we have so far. Sexuality is a path to learning this. It makes perfect sense to me that sexuality and its inherent power has been silenced, suppressed, cajoled and repulsed, for it is the root of our lifeforce. A mindset that creates a culture of death and violence cannot allow a vital lifeforce to direct individuals. Awaken the hidden potential of your G-spot and female ejaculation with the following exercise.

EXERCISE: ACCESSING THE EROTIC SPIRITUAL REALM

No alcohol, marijuana or drugs of any kind are to be used at least 72 hours before this exercise.

Find a wilderness setting in warm, sunny weather by a creek or a warm, moonlit evening, with or without a fire. A private, quiet, outdoor setting is essential for this as you are about to access higher consciousness. Bring a cock ring or cock-and-ball strap for him and Ben-Wa balls or preferably a finished gemstone that is golfball-sized for her. Bring a thick, padded blanket and two pillows, a charcoal burner and sage and frankincense. Bring an icon of your choice, perhaps Isis, Lilith, Shiva, Pan or the Horned God. Bring a journal or sketch pad, chocolate, and water. Bring matches.

Remove your clothes. Light the incense and sage. Smudge the smoke of the lit sage over your bodies to lighten up your energy and purify it of negative thoughts and emotions. Look into each other's eyes as you cleanse and prepare each other with the sage. Put on the cock ring and insert the stone ball into the vagina. Then say this centring prayer or one of your choice: 'Let this sacred act be protected by the gods. Let this sacred act of love fly in the wind in gratitude to that which gives us life. Let this sacred act in which we are about to partake nourish us and all energy around us.'Sit face to face, hold hands and cross your legs around each other in a comfortable position. Meditate on the feelings that arise in your body. Say this and repeat it ten times, very slowly like a mantra: 'Pleasure is love and I am opening to pleasure. Pleasure is love and I am opening to pleasure. Pleasure is love and I am opening to pleasure.' Allow your body to express its physical sensations and stay 'present', that is, fully aware of them. Meditate on the sensations that well up, such as in your chest or stomach or loins. Move if a part of your body wants to move. Let it lead as you keep the mind focused on the mantra, and the body's voice of feeling and movement talking to you. The practice is about having complete trust in the process, and in the guidance you are receiving through your body.

Now, touch his perineum and her nipples with your fingertips, very gently, and do not move or stroke. Meditate on giving and receiving only love as you do this, and on the pleasure you receive by the contact. Say over and over again 'This is what love feels like. This is what love feels like. This is what love feels like.' Remember to move your touch imperceptibly at first until you zero in on the love feelings. Then, increase the sensation of touch ever so slightly. Whenever the love feeling goes away and gets replaced with the urge to satisfy the erotic sensations, stop all stimulation and contact.

Recentre and refocus on the love feeling and start again. Each time you will get further pleasuring each other before you have to quit to refocus on the love feeling. After six times or so of stopping and starting, depending on your experience and ability to hold focus and pleasure and love, you have made it to the point where the G-spot is massaged.

Here is the point at which the G-spot can be truly awakened to its full potential, as the gateway to intense physical sensations of love, deep-seated emotions and mystical states of consciousness. Keep massaging the spots – either he or she is likely to be receiving the massage, although it is possible for both to give and receive at the same time. Stop whenever the pleasure cascades over into sensations of lust, and then begin again when one has recentred on the love feeling.

Always begin slowly at first. Let sensations and emotions surface and acknowledge them with this holy greeting 'I welcome you. You are the truth in me. Be voiced.' If at any time emotions have to be expressed or the intimacy becomes too intense and uncomfortable for you, simply stop. Express the emotions with your partner witnessing and listening only. Or, end the session with the prayer outlined below. If not, continue. Come into union with this erotic, devotional love prayer: 'I receive from you pure love and return its healing energy with joy.' Each person repeats this three times. Lie (or sit) entwined and keep turning the feelings of pleasure into love.

Remember to discontinue all movement if the sensations of love get lost to the sexual urge. Eye contact is essential. You will at some point enter orgasmic bliss completely enveloped in this feeling of love, or the erotic love feelings will dissipate into a feeling of full satisfaction as if you had orgasmed. Either way will be utterly divine.

Afterward, you may notice you are in an altered state of consciousness. You can tell this by a heightened sense of hearing, sight or other sensory awareness. Commune with nature, experiment with breathing with the trees or listen to the rocks or wind. This is where the practice ends and where your personal experience and path begin. You are on your own, finding your own truth, using your union with your partner to become one with the other beings around you.

In a half-hour to an hour-and-a-half, you will regain your usual sense of reality. End the session with sage smudge and a prayer of gratitude to the cosmos and to each other. Eat the chocolate and finish the water. Write down your impressions of the experience or sketch them. Snuggle up and nap or go to sleep for the evening. This entire erotic meditation can be done without a partner with oneself. Allow three hours.

DOLORES FRENCH

A little way out, a little way in

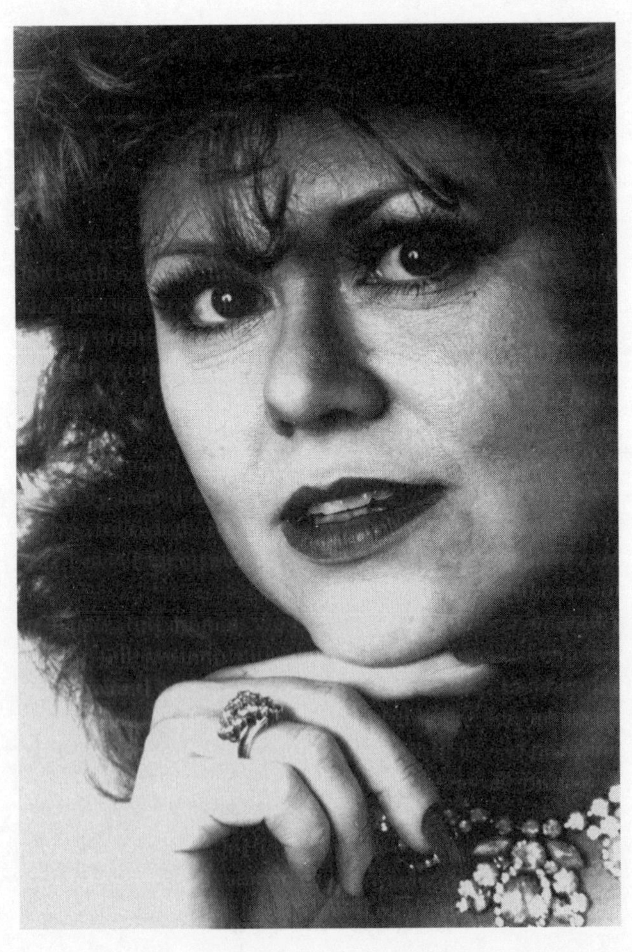

Dolores French was born in 1951 in Kentucky, US. She studied journalism and photography and eventually moved into radio, working in the managerial section of a radio station.

She has worked as a prostitute all around the world. After all the travelling she has done she loves being at home, in Georgia, US and her work consists of phone sex, specialising in domination. She also writes for Hustler *magazine.*

Dolores is presently working on a couple of books, has a column in the magazines Vixen *and* The Scene, *and is a regular television and radio commentator on the sex industry.*

I still work as a prostitute and have regular clients that I have been seeing for twenty years. If I go for a week without seeing anyone, it's not good as I really enjoy my work. I never want to retire. I see the way I work now as different from when I first started because I am more comfortable with myself.

I feel very comfortable with my body and I find that men are grateful to be with someone who is sexual and skilled. Men are not as critical of women's bodies as women are. Sexually I am so much better now than when I was in my twenties. I remember when I was in my twenties I worked with a woman who was in her late forties or early fifties, and I knew then that I would never be as sexy as she was until I reached her age. She had a sensuality and artistic approach to sexuality, and she was so graceful in her approach. I have a sexiness now that I could not have had earlier in my life.

I have many relationships in my life, which are both sexual and non-sexual. Many people find the relationship I have with my husband is odd, but I would not have involved myself with him to begin with if he were not open to the person that I am. I would advise a couple who want to introduce other people into their relationship to be open and honest and really understand what the boundaries and commitments of your relationship arc.

Being very clear does not mean cornering your partner into an agreement on how to operate the relationship that is not really in their heart. If I were to make an agreement with my husband to have a monogamous relationship it would never work, because that is not in my heart. Being upfront and honest about that is so important. Sex is such a small part of a whole relationship and expecting it to be the thing that either holds a relationship together or dissolves it I think is stupid.

When addressing the issue of monogamy at the International Conference On Prostitution, zoologist Robin Baker told us that human sperm is specialised. Perhaps fourteen different types of guys in there are each doing a very specialised task, one of which is to kill. Baker proposed that these sperm have been genetically programmed to assassinate others because they expect to find other sperm from other males in any given vagina.

Baker also pondered an interesting observation on the shape of the penis. Why is that 'tip' there anyway? Apparently, Baker says, it is to act as a plunger to suck out the other guy's sperm in the built-in `back and forth, in and out' motion.

Recently I have been considering plastic surgery and after a visit to a specialist I had an insight into the physically beneficial effects of the years of professional oral sex I had been performing. I put pen to paper to record my feelings about this.

My face has fallen and it can't get up

Pink. When I was walking down the hallway I expected I was in the right place when I saw a pinkish glow pulsing from the end of the corridor. Then I saw figures – people, moving behind huge etched glass double doors. They were all wearing pink outfits. Scrubs. And nurses' smocks. Surgical caps. All pink.

It wasn't crowded. I was glad to see that no-one looked perfect, but no-one looked hideous either – no accidents waiting to be reconstructed. Cosmetic surgery. 'We really are all grown-ups now,' I thought. I wanted them to just take me in and fix everything, adjust everything, 'while I'm unconscious, and spit me out in a few days all reworked'.

Then I went in to see the doctor, Rod Hester. He looked like he could use a bit of his own medicine, but I felt comfortable that he had chosen otherwise – at least I hope that was the case.

I explained that I just wanted my chin and eyes tucked. I understood before I got there that a little chin tuck might be necessary. Then he started showing me how they would restore my whole face. It was impressive. He did it all with his fingers, not one of those computer-imaging things. I think the computer-imaging things are fun, but I'm suspicious of the results – after all, Fred Astaire dances with a Broom-vac via computer imaging. Besides, I've got plenty of images of where different parts of my face used to be – they are called photographs. Anyway, with just his fingers he was able to put all the pieces back to where they once were.

It gave me nostalgic longings, sentimental memories of tight elasticity. Gone are the days when fellatio held my flesh tight in place on my face. As Rod poked at my jaws and jowls, and speculated about restoring cheekbone definition, I wondered if maybe doing a six-week stint sucking cocks in the Caribbean couldn't do the same thing. This is something I can't stop thinking about – the physical benefits of cheap whorehouse life. I was in great condition when I worked those places.

Back in the 1980s I wrote about fellatio: 'If I didn't do it every day my tongue got tired, my jaws got tired, my lips got tired. When I went home for a little rest and recreation in Atlanta, however, everyone commented about how the structure of my face seemed to have changed. My cheeks seemed leaner, my jawline tighter. I knew it was from giving head.'Anyway, back here in the slash and suck world of cosmetic surgery Rod was doing a good job of showing me he could cut here and tuck there and suck a little out right here and inject it there and in about six hours make my face as good as new, almost. A mini brow-lift would be the crowning touch.

I could see that he was right, though I never lost sight of the benefits that blow jobs could have. Still, I could see that while the fellatio treatment could cure a lot of ailments, surgery was the only solution to some of the problems.

Now it was time to see the appointment secretary, Libby, about scheduling all this and paying for it. She was a cute young woman with a cute even-younger nose. After all her figuring, including the overnight stay in the recovery suite, Libby announced the total cost would be (are you ready for your own mini brow-lift?) US$14,025! Libby immediately added that, in my case, the mini brow-lift might not be absolutely necessary, bringing the cost down to about $12,000.

Is it bestiality or professional animal breeding? Who decides these things? Or, my face has fallen and it can't get up. I have a spare $15,000 for cosmetic surgery. I have a spare $15,000 for cosmetic surgery. 'I have a spare $15,000 for cosmetic surgery' became my daily affirmation.

Health insurance doesn't cover such procedures, I'm told. Who decides these things? A guy who smokes cigarettes gets emphysema, and the insurance company covers his medical costs! He could live with that breathing problem. His death certificate is no more likely to read 'Cause of death: emphysema' than mine will read 'gravity'. But can I get my share of medical care? No! Because some alcoholic executive is sucking up all the medical insurance money treating his liver ailments. Let him turn yellow! While I'm doing no more than walking around upright on this planet, I'm being victimised by gravity! If falling flesh doesn't count as an accident, who decides what does? Maybe the same nitwits who lobby legislation defining the difference between bestiality and professional animal breeding. What brilliant philosopher proposed that it's legal to jerk-off dogs, horses etc. as long as it's for profit, but it's illegal if it's just good fun for all involved? I want a head count of the elected idiots that voted this professional dog-pimping into law. There's no doubt in my mind that it's the same bunch of befuddled people who came up with these health insurance coverage policies.

If you can spare $15,000 for my beautification/historical restoration project email Frenchdom@aol.com. Donations are not tax deductible.

EXERCISE: GIVING THE BEST BLOW JOB

I perfected the best way to do a blow job in the Caribbean. The women I worked with used to sit around waiting for our next client, each discussing the best method to suck a guy off in the least possible time. Some believed that you should suck hard, or that tongue flicks were the answer, others thought deep throat or using an up-and-down speed was it. Another woman believed that placing a finger in the anus made it the best while another was adamant it was all the moaning-and-slurping sound effects that made it. I tried each of these methods, realising that none was the answer but when I put them all together and found my own natural rhythm the men found it amazingly exciting.

I learned a lot from the way Japanese men make love. They don't just go in and out, they make a pattern of it. They go in, a little way out, a little way in, a little way out, a little out, a little out, way in, in, in. I took this rhythm into the way I did blow jobs as I teased, stroked and added a sudden surprise of tickling as the man relaxed into deep pleasure. I got rave reviews from clients and a lot of repeat business and found that it didn't usually take longer than seven minutes for my clients to come.

8

Film and Pornography

Hollywood movies of the 1990s show more sex than ever before; explicit lovemaking scenes, masturbation and even homoerotic encounters are no longer uncommon. Television portrayals of sexuality are also increasingly explicit, with the high-rating soap operas showing (or at least implying) not just sexy encounters between married couples, but also casual affairs, sex between strangers and even the odd *ménage-a-trois*. It's a long way from *Leave it to Beaver*.

The amount of visual sexual information people see is so high that when they purchase an X-rated video for personal use it is not surprising they want even more explicit imagery. The video porn industry is relatively new, only as old as the video recorder itself, so people's ability to buy or hire porn movies for private use is historically a new phenomenon. The home video recorder has also allowed people to star in their own erotic escapades. The X-rated video industry has burgeoned and in the US the Kinsey Institute estimated that one in three videos rented is X-rated.

In a typical X-rated video the focus is on genital action, not on the storyline or emotional interplay between the characters. Women have long been critical of the X-rated video industry, to the point of running campaigns to have them banned or claiming that they contribute to violence against women, including rape. Other women have not accepted that explicit porn causes violence, but have still been critical of the way women's sexual pleasure is frequently ignored, and they are often portrayed in demeaning ways. In fairness, while pornography can be said to reflect the views of society, including stereotypical views of women, it cannot be blamed for creating them.

Free speech activists, some of whom are also feminists, have argued that censorship is not the answer. Rather, women taking some degree of control within the industry is. They claim that there is an eager market for sexually explicit adult films from women and couples, markets that have been traditionally ignored. They argue that films can be sexually hot, yet reflect a new progressive view of women who are in charge of their sexuality and their lives.

By the mid-1980s this theory was put into practice. Independent erotic video-makers started producing porn for women, couples and lesbian porn for lesbians. And it sold. Former porn star Candida Royalle swapped places for a starring role on the other side of the lens and produced a best-selling string of movies for women and couples. The independent publishers of lesbian sex magazine *On Our Backs* launched a video line, Fatale Films. These video companies continue and have gone from strength to strength. Other independent female video companies produced new-style erotica and the old boys' porn network eventually caught on and started producing videos for the couples market.

The popularity of the new porn produced by companies run by women has shown that this is the direction of the future. The videos they produce contain nudity and graphic depictions of sex, but no coercion or violence. They also place emphasis on a woman's sexual pleasure and give a realistic depiction of women's sexuality. Although these new porn pioneers have less capital than the mainstream producers, they spend up to ten times more on their films.

Women are also at the forefront of another type of erotic video: sex education videos that show and describe what makes sex better, without erotic titillation. When women started exploring the G-spot and female ejaculation it became obvious that there was only so far you could go without explicit visual explanation. The same video porn pioneers produced the new sex education videos, which proved to have the same eager audience. Videos on female ejaculation, Tantric sex, anal pleasure for men and safe sex for women and couples were eagerly sought for their no-nonsense, sex-positive approach – and their sense of humour.

Women who work within the porn industry are now less closeted about their professions than previously, with stars such as Nina Hartley making the cross-over to Hollywood in the film *Boogie Nights*. They have set up support systems for each other and created a new-style sisterhood within the sex industry. The development of women's visual imagery, including video, has been an essential component of women's sexual empowerment. It is a way of duplicating what they see in the best relationships, from how to seduce someone to how you touch and caress a lover.

Statistics of porn video rentals show that people frequently seek out erotic material that is outside their sexual preference. So straight women hire movies of gay men, lesbians hire those depicting bisexual menage-a-trois and straight men (famously) hire lesbian videos more than almost any other kind. Every survey shows that while some regard society as becoming more conservative, a large percentage of the general public want the right to have sexually explicit material available to consenting adults in their own home. Video sales show that the popularity of porn is not waning.

Despite the political and legal battles that continue around classification and censorship many personal issues remain for couples who wish to enjoy X-rated videos together. Many people feel embarrassed to bring up their desire to watch a porn video with their partner; some fear that letting their partner know what they fantasise about exposes their sexual vulnerability. Others worry that the exoticism of the on-screen scenario compares unfavourably with their own domesticity. Beautiful porn stars can cause partners to feel uneasy about their own body, and those with impossible endowments can also cause anxiety.

In this chapter Nan Kinney addresses this and shows you how to have a romantic porn video date, while Candida Royalle and Nina Hartley reveal what life is really like in the sex industry.

CANDIDA ROYALLE

Fantasies: a reflection of what is happening in our life

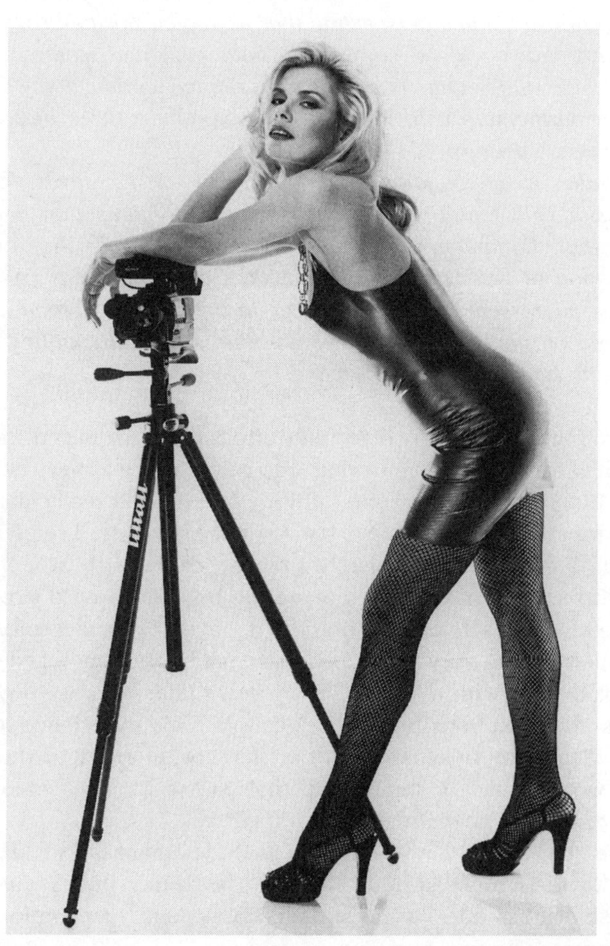

Candida Royalle, a native New Yorker, comes from a background rich in the arts with training in art, music, voice and dance. Her educational background includes the New York High School of Arts and Design, Parson's School of Design and the City University of New York.

In San Francisco, she became active in the avant-garde theatre scene, performing with the infamous Cockettes, the Angels of Light and the late Divine. She later moved on to sing in jazz clubs and classical choruses. It was in San Francisco, in the more liberal 1970s, that Ms Royalle turned to working in X-rated movies for additional income.

In 1984 she founded Femme Productions in order to create erotic films from a woman's perspective that promoted positive sexual role-modelling that could be enjoyed by both men and women. Twelve movies later, the Femme line is now distributed worldwide by PHE Inc, who, in partnership with Royalle, will co-produce three new Femme features each year.

Royalle is a founding board member of Feminists for Free Expression (FFE), a non-profit, anti-censorship organisation. She is the only 'adult' filmmaker to have been invited to join the American Association of Sex Educators, Councillors and Therapists (AASECT). She has addressed many conferences in the US and abroad and has appeared on many major talk shows. She is currently writing a book on female sexual self-empowerment.

At a young age I use to draw and often it was of naked men and women with a story behind what was going on. I was very sensually aware but I didn't fool around until my late teens. I really liked boys and from an early age I had a strong sense of touch. I remember at thirteen having a friend I use to practise dance with, which would turn into a game of one of us being the boy who would slowly run our hands up each other's bodies. It never became genital but I remember feeling very excited and sensual by the touch and smell. I did not do this with a boy for many years later because boys were always intent on your breasts or genitals. This experience inspired me to display more sensuality in my movies, in order to show men what women like. I duplicated that scene in my video *Three Daughters* with two eighteen-year-old girls.

The new video I am working on at the moment is *Eyes of Desire*. This movie is more serious than the last ones that I have done because it looks into voyeurism and obsessions. I am exploring the idea that sometimes you can get drawn to someone in a way that becomes more of an obsession than a healthy relationship. This reflects quite a change in my work. My earlier movies were quite safe? I made them 'soft' because it was a new area for women to explore fantasies. Now my work has become more explicit, certainly not in the traditional hard-core sense, like when men direct erotic films.

I think women are ready for more: they like seeing men's erections, they like seeing the lovemaking, but I still don't have those come shots all over the place. The other thing that has changed is the exploration of fantasy, and the whole delicious aspect of surrender and letting go into your desires and letting your lover dominate you.

When I was a porn star I enjoyed being in front of the camera dressing up and playing roles, but the most difficult part for me was engaging in sex in front of the camera. I am not an exhibitionist, in fact, I am a modest person. I worked in the golden age of porn – for 35 mm high-budget films then, you had to audition and learn lines. This does not happen any more. As a young struggling artist it was a way of making a lot of money quickly. I prefer being behind the camera, I love creating the script, shooting it and being in control of the images. I wish I had worked for someone like me when I was an actress, instead of traditional porn movie-makers. When I audition I look for people who bring character and personality to the part they are playing, as well as being able to let go and explore their own eroticism and sensuality. I don't want people who have done so much formulaic work that they just follow the typical porno rules. It is a difficult job because you have to take on a role and act it out, and become erotic while still playing the role of that person.

When I was working as a porn actress and showed up on the set, the director or producer would be sleazy and not really care what they were doing. It made me feel cheap about what I was doing. But when they took an interest and were creative and innovative it made me feel good and I was able to give more to the role. I approach my actresses and actors in the same way. I am very serious about what I do, and I want us to enjoy ourselves as well as produce a product that they can feel proud of. I expect a lot of professionalism from them and in return I give them a comfortable and respectful set to work in.

When I can I always use real-life couples because they bring with them a certain amount of added heat. My second choice is to find couples who are really hot for one another. I look for chemistry between people. I like creating a positive environment for people to work in and I have a lot of respect for them because they are making themselves very vulnerable.

Safer sex practices and condoms were introduced into my movies in 1987 and in *Taste of Ambrosia* there is a very sexy scene of a woman putting a black condom on her partner. In *Sensual Escapes* we deal with how to bring up the subject of safe sex and I have a safe sex message at the end of the videos.

I see the future of erotic films becoming more and more of a blend of what women and men are looking for as we grow together. I have started a trend of showing more of what women want sexually and depicting more sensuality in the sex. Showing the build-up is important, as is the storyline. Men watching these movies are paying attention to what it is that women like and responding to them and enjoying the experience at the same time. As women become more comfortable watching these movies they are open to seeing things that are more racy or explicit.

To maintain the excitement in our relationships we are looking for more fantasy role-play and ideas. This is reflected in the how-to or entertaining adult movies. The feedback I receive from men watching my videos is that they love seeing their wives getting excited, which turns them on. Many men tell me they don't like hard-core porn and therefore find the videos very sensual. Women get ideas from the videos to take into their life.

I had a young woman staying at my place when I was away who watched my videos and she told me that they opened a new area of possibilities for her. She had been in a relationship for four years which was not very experimental or communicative. Through the inspiration she received from my videos she was able to try out new things, which were great hits. She learned these new techniques from watching the movies, not by being promiscuous, and this made her feel comfortable about her desires.

Over the years I have done dance, yoga, callisthenics and weights. This enables me to clear my mind. The script for *Eyes of Desire* came from me working out, wondering if anyone could see me, which I adapted into a story of a woman at home with a high-powered telescope. The twist is that not only does she start getting curious about observing others, but that she is being observed.

Fantasies are a reflection of what is happening in our life. For me I have to constantly be in a powerful position of running my own company, and I know there is nothing more delicious than giving up that control. Also I believe that the basis of our fantasies comes from our upbringing and how sexuality was presented to us when we were growing up.

I come from a Catholic background where sex was forbidden fruit and you should not go there – you had to save yourself. For a lot of women I feel this has instilled a sense of shame and guilt about our sexuality. Therefore to lose control and have an orgasm and receive pleasure we have to pretend we are being forced to give up that control. This is what gives rise to the 'rape' fantasy – we obviously don't want to be raped in real life, but we need a trigger that gives us permission to receive pleasure and give up control.

A wonderful sexual thing to do in a relationship is to write your fantasy to your lover, leave him or her a secret note, or read to him or her a story that you have read from an erotic novel. Once you have shared your fantasies together there is nothing sexier than to speak your partner's favourite fantasy out loud, while he or she either pleasures himself or herself or you do. Fantasy is not necessarily something you act out. I was in a monogamous relationship where we would fantasise about each other being with someone else, but in real life we were very possessive and jealous. However, we would talk about it and make believe, which was very positive for us and a great way to play.

EXERCISE: MAKING YOUR OWN HOME MOVIES

Watching movies opens you up, gives you ideas and gets you in touch with inner fantasies that you might not have been aware of. Self-pleasuring as you watch erotic videos is a very good way to feel connected with your fantasies without judging them.

Making your own home movies can be sexy and fun, but I believe couples should put a lot of thought into whether it's a good idea for them. There is always the possibility of the video being found and circulated. Personally I never let myself be photographed or videoed in a sexual situation, as I am now a very private person.

One way to have the fun of making your own erotic home video without actually making a video is to use a camera recorder without any film in it hooked up to a TV monitor. This way while you are being 'filmed' making love you can watch yourself and your partner on the TV. This can be very exciting.

NAN KINNEY

Pornography: expanding our sexual horizons

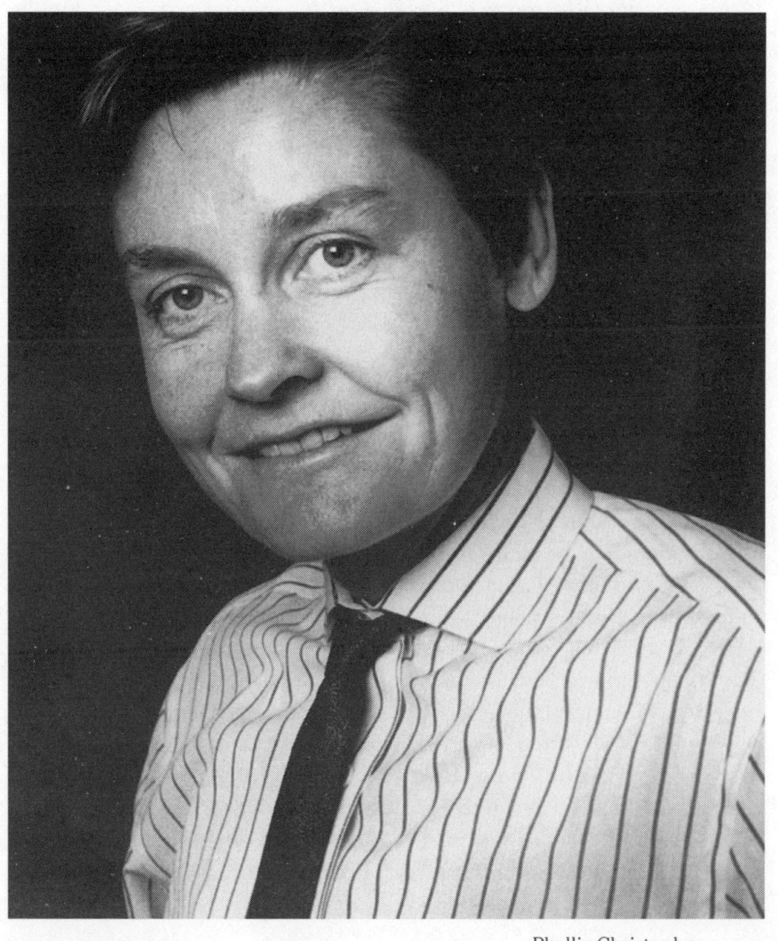

Phyllis Christopher

Nan Kinney is the producer of Fatale videos and one of the founding publishers of the highly acclaimed and notorious magazine, On Our Backs. A native of Austin, Minnesota, she began her foray into the world of lesbian pornography in the early 1980s when she moved to San Francisco to check out the SM scene.

When she realised that there was no venue for lesbian sexual imagery made by and for lesbians, she and two partners, Deborah Sundahl and Susie Bright, solicited material and published their first issue of On Our Backs *in June 1984. With the success and popularity of the magazine, Nan and Deborah jumped into videos.*

In January 1985, they released Private Pleasures *and* Shadows, *two videos that starred real-life lesbian lovers and presented for the first time sexually explicit footage made by and for lesbians. Later titles included* Suburban Dykes, Safe is Desire, How to Female Ejaculate, Hungry Hearts *and* Burlezk Live I & II.

By 1994, with On Our Backs being published bimonthly and the circulation at an all-time high, Nan and Deborah decided to sell the magazine and pursue their separate interests.

Nan now runs Fatale Videos full-time and has expanded the company's mission to include bisexual pornographic images. A recent release, Bend Over Boyfriend, *starring sex educators Carol Queen and Robert Morgan, addresses women giving men anal pleasure. Currently in production is* Rev Her Up, *a fun-filled lesbian urban romp through the back rooms of an auto-repair shop.*

Nan's goal has always been to present alternative images of sexuality and she has now expanded the goal to include bisexual images. She believes that sex is an important part of people's lives, and women, and lesbians in particular, have always been portrayed in a very limited way in traditional pornography. She wants people to have other images of themselves as a way to burst out of the ingrained images in mainstream porn.

The inspiration for *On Our Backs* came from the fact that there was no porn for lesbians. We went to a book shop, trying to find some porn, and all we found was one book, which was fine, but I wanted more. They didn't even have *The Story of O.* I always liked pornography, I always liked to read *Playboy* and *Penthouse*, and I wanted something authentic, a magazine made by and for lesbians. I wanted to produce something that more realistically represented my sexuality as a butch lesbian.

I wasn't alone in this desire for sexually explicit images of lesbians. All my friends were taking pictures of one another and didn't have a place to publish them. We knew there was a need. We wanted it, so we figured other people wanted it too. This was in 1984, the time of the sex wars in the lesbian community, when lesbians were marching at the frontlines of the anti-porn movement with Andrea Dworkin and Catherine MacKinnon.

On the flip side of that were these sexually active, radical lesbians who thought sex was great and pornography was a viable way to explore our sexuality together, to expand our sexual horizons. Obviously, I was part of the latter group. We did it as sort of a political move in the beginning, not a business move, as a great way of fighting back at the anti-porn feminists, and making a statement for pro-sex lesbians, many of whom also considered themselves feminists.

I literally had been in bed with women who wouldn't let me penetrate them because it wasn't politically correct. It pissed me off that the feminist political bullshit had infiltrated these women's sex lives. They were denying themselves pleasure because of it. It also was a very special time in San Francisco in 1984, a creative time. Politics was the glue that brought us together. We wanted to make our mark on the world.

The lesbian community's reaction to the first issue of *On Our Backs* was totally overwhelming – either for or against, a very strong reaction. We got hate mail. We got people in our faces calling us Nazis at San Francisco's Gay Pride where we had a booth. But it was more overwhelmingly positive than negative. 'Thank God!' they'd say. 'Finally something I can relate to and get off on!' We got enough support to publish more issues. People sent us submissions for the magazine – erotic stories and pictures came pouring in from all over the country.

Some of the artists and writers were already established, such as Tee Corrine, Lee Lynch, Joan Nestle, Dorothy Allison, Pat Califia, for example. Others essentially started their erotic publishing careers off with *On Our Backs*, for instance, photographers Morgan Gwenwald, Honey Lee Cotrell, Phyllis Christopher, Jill Posner, and fiction writers such as Jewell Gomez.

Because *On Our Backs* got such attention we realised there were other ways to produce porn. It was natural. We wanted to be the Mitchell Brothers (owners of the well-known San Francisco O'Farrell

Theater, a strip club, and producers of videos) of the lesbian porn world. It was fun! We had a great time. We also began to make some money at this time.

Women loved it. For example, the women-only strip show, Burlezk, ran sold-out weekly shows for four years. At that time there were no existing distributors for the types of videos we did – we had to sell them ourselves through direct mail and advertising in On Our Backs. Once again, response was overwhelming. Our mailbag was full every day. We'd get letters that were very explicit from readers and viewers. They'd say, 'I want to see more hairy butches', or 'Thanks for your images of big women. Let's see more'. So we knew we were on the right track.

Now I'm strictly in the video business and focusing on producing and selling Fatale videos. There are more distributors now that will carry the videos. I'm thinking of Good Vibrations in particular, but also lesbian and gay friendly video companies around the country. I've expanded the subject matter to include bisexual women's point of view, because there is nothing really made for them either.

You can find videos with two guys and a girl, but that's not the same. Our latest release is *Bend Over Boyfriend*, an informative tape about how to pleasure your man anally, which I believe is the first of its kind. It's selling like mad and during the year has frequently been the number one best-selling video for Good Vibrations. This tells me there is a need for this type of imagery.

My life really hasn't changed because of that era. I'm the same person. I'm still a lesbian pornographer, which is what I always wanted to be when I grew up. One of my biggest role models was Larry Flynt. Also Hugh Hefner, the Mitchell Brothers, Gloria Steinem, Joani Blank (founder of Good Vibrations) – these people were my role models. I'm still following the goals I had at that time.

I've always seen myself on the outside of things culturally, sexually, politically. I'm a daredevil. I don't have any preconceived notions of how my life should be. I'm willing to try different things. In the 1980s I explored SM because at that time those were the only lesbians talking about sex. Or even practising it, doing it. I was curious, and I had the opportunity to explore it, but I learned it doesn't get me off that much. I learned that it's not the SM I'm into as much as being open around sex in general, my sexuality around butch and femme, that sort of thing.

I'm the same person I was sexually, that I was in high school, but

I'm more at ease with myself now. I'm a Taurus, I'm a butch who likes femmes. I've explored a lot of things but I've come back to the fact that this is what my sexuality is. I'm your basic meat-and-potatoes butch. I like a girlfriend, I like a house, I like my work. I'm not that different from most people. It's just that my work is producing sexual images, which puts me outside the American mainstream. Also I have had the bonus of having better sex because of my job.

I want more of the same for the future. Back to the future, if you will. For as long as I'm able, I want to be a producer of pornography. I'd like to be able to bring somebody up in the business and let them have it. I want to work and encourage young women coming into the porn business, to be a mentor of young women, and lesbians in particular.

Presently, my video *Rev Her Up* is in the works. I'm trying for the first time to put humour and sex together. Can people really laugh when they have sex? When they're turned on? Does laughter turn them on? I have a gut feeling I know, from all the times I've laughed in bed that we can hit that spot with a video. Having just relocated to New York, I've put together a different team of women and men to work on this. Even though it will be a lesbian video, we'll have men in minor roles in the video because men, gay men especially, are in our lives.

The other thing we're doing is to further explore international sales and distribution of all our titles. We've still got difficulty in some countries with censorship. This is an age-old issue. From the start of my career, fighting censorship has been part of my job, part of the essential work I have to do. In the beginning it was censorship within the lesbian community and now I'm dealing with censorship on an international level.

The Internet offers a potential solution to some of this, but you still have to mail your product into countries, and the stores cannot display it. Even in New York City this is happening under the mayor's plan to turn the city into one big Disneyworld. On the Internet we can display what we've got. It's a great frontier, although we don't know how it's going to turn out, especially with pending American legislation that would limit what's available on the Internet.

TIPS: ROSES, VODKA AND VIDEOTAPE - HOW TO WATCH A PORN MOVIE

As with any sort of sexual foreplay, watching dirty movies together with your partner doesn't always work. You usually can't just pick one off the shelf, pop it in the VCR, sit back and expect to get randy. (Unless, of course, you're already randy and the video is really just the signal to make love, like adjusting the lighting or putting on some sexy music.) Porn videos as foreplay takes some forethought. Here's my advice on the subject.

Assuming you're looking to a porn video as part of the seduction or turn-on, I find the biggest pitfall is expecting too much from an erotic or porn video. People who haven't watched a lot of porn are often surprised and disappointed at the low production quality, poor scripts, bad acting and the general formulaic, juvenile and male-orientated content. This disappointment can be a true turn-off. So the most important thing I have to say about watching porn is: be forgiving.

Try to find one thing in a video that turns you on. If you can find even that one thing, I think the video is a success. Maybe it's a certain camera angle that lets you see what it looks like from your partner's point of view when she's fucking you. Maybe it's a look in one of the actresses' eyes, a stance, a sentence, an orgasmic scream, anything that sends a twitch to your clit and that you can hold onto for later fantasies.

Learning how to appreciate porn can take time. Be patient. Do it with your partner. Rent a lot of tapes until you find the ones that arouse you, and think about what it is you like about it so you can hone in on the types of porn you should be getting. Talk about it with your partner - maybe you'll find you like different sorts of porn. For example, I think of porn videos like I think of action movies: some sort of plot is needed, but it's really all about the action, the sex. I have my favourite action heroes (Arnold Schwarzenegger, Linda

Hamilton) and I have my favourite porn heroes (Sharon Mitchell, Nina Hartley). Usually I can watch anything they do and get into it.

So once you've found some porn you like, make an evening of it! Have a video date - buy your honey some roses, have a little vodka (or beverage of your choice), wear something you feel sexy in. Bring out your collection of porn videos, or get something new (but within your pre-determined rating of potential for turn-on). Get comfortable - no phones, no kids, no neighbours. Let the tape roll and the juices will flow.

NINA HARTLEY

Sex-positivism

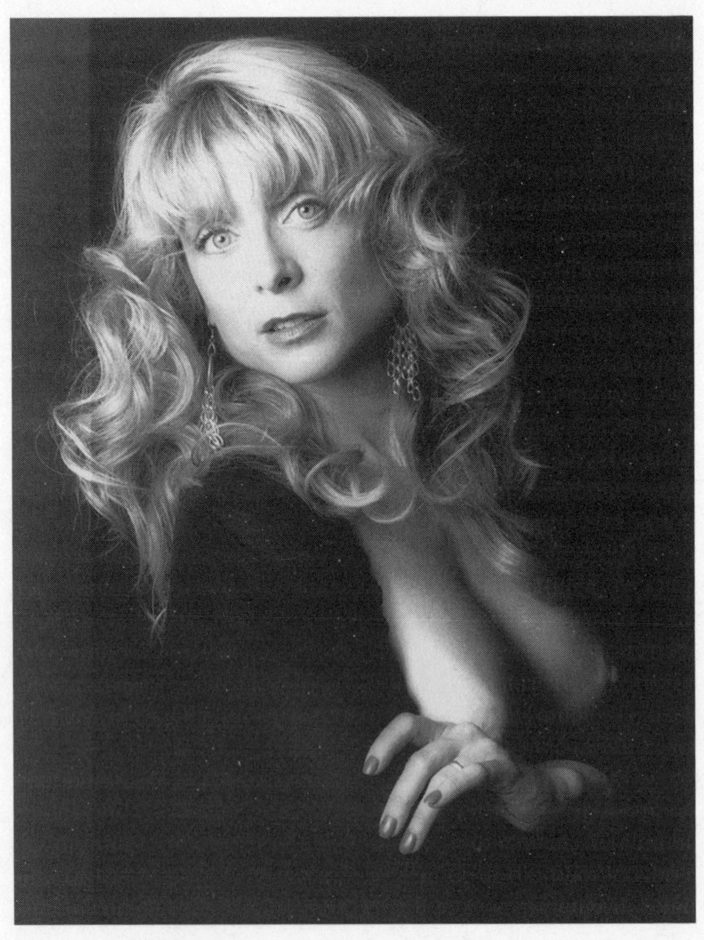

Nina Hartley, RN, is a fifteen-year veteran of 'adult' videos. She is a dancer, educator, director, actress, advocate, activist, writer and swinger. One of the most vocal of the sex-positive feminists who came on the scene in the mid-1980s, she is tireless in promoting her sexual philosophy, a unique synthesis of science, humanism, feminism, socialism and personal responsibility. A charismatic and engaging speaker, she is popular with a wide range of audiences.

After starting as a dancer while going to nursing school in California, Nina found she liked the explicit medium enough to make the transition. In 1985, after graduating magna cum laude, she went full-time into the movies. She has been the winner of most of the porn industry's most prestigious awards, and she continues to act, as well as produce, direct and write her own videos. She lives with her husband, Dave, and her wife, Bobby, in a long-standing ménage-a-trois in Berkeley, California, US.

I was one of the first women to declare myself a feminist porn star and this now represents my abiding love of women (and by extension, men) in all its manifestations. It obligates me to engage the world, to share my knowledge with interested people and to champion the cause of sex positivism in an otherwise hostile environment. It is because of my passionate sex-positive feminism that I find the energy to engage 'the enemy' in dialogue rather than shut them out. It is a statement of self-love that does not come at the expense of others; instead, it is at the service of others.

Initially, I publicly identified as a feminist because I believed in the principles of gender equality and wanted to promote them. I wanted to bring a feminist eye to the inner workings of commercial pornography, not just read theoretical treatises on the evils of objectification. If sexual self-determination was every woman's birthright and if my body was truly mine, then I concluded there was no reason that I could not conduct myself with feminist-inspired self-respect within the world of sex work.

Frankly, I also did it to make myself more interesting to journalists and scholars and to lead them in my direction as someone who was willing to speak to them. At the time, I was one of the few performers who were willing to talk to 'outsiders' about the business. While feminists were talking about porn, few were talking to the people who made it. Fewer still were involved in making it.

In general, feminists felt themselves better than 'those women' who were willing to subjugate themselves to such an exploitative industry. Their arrogance permitted them to ignore sex workers' stories and summarily dismiss what they had to say. Well, I was of their class and educational background, so they would not be able to dismiss me easily. I wanted to be an articulate defender of sexually-orientated material and of consensual sexual behaviour, no matter how 'kinky' it seemed to the uninitiated.

I try to keep my family life separate from my work. My husband is intensely private, and I honour that. My wife, Bobby, and I would have more of an open-door policy with regards to friends and the media. Out of respect for his sensibilities we limit the people we allow into our home. Instead, we go to their place. There are certain areas that are not totally open for discussion during interviews. Because my public persona is very closely aligned with my 'real' self, there is very little problem for me in making the transition from 'in public' to 'at home'.

I tend to form relationships with other sex-positive people: we all love to talk shop! The discussions we have are very exciting. With fans, I expect a lot of sexual talk, but I don't normally discuss any 'trials and tribulations' with them although I love any opportunity to share my sexual journey with interested viewers or readers. As a self-identified, out exhibitionist, the satisfactory expression of my sexuality depends in part on it being 'public', that is, enjoyed by others as entertainment or education. When it comes to the most deeply personal emotional experiences, I must first experience them in private before I can think of translating them to the screen or stage.

I am now fifteen years into my career and I produce, direct and star in a successful line of sex education videos, from which I receive a royalty (one of the first performers to do so). I am starting to make inroads into 'straight' projects, most notably a part in the 1997 film *Boogie Nights*. I'm increasing my profile as a lecturer, advocate, educator and pundit, in addition to 'merely' being an entertainer. As always, I mentor novice performers and provide a sympathetic ear for people with sexual problems.

My work has changed as I've matured and become more experienced as a performer. What has remained the same is my dedication to showcasing empowered, positive, female sexuality. I've always tried to be an accessible role model for women who are developing their own sexual identities. Now, I just have a bigger venue for it.

I see myself working as an actress for as long as I want. As the boomers age, they (especially the women) desire and deserve to see themselves represented on screen as viable, sexy people. Performers my age can only benefit from this unique demographic phenomenon. Fans tend to be fans for life: if nothing else, their adoration alone will guarantee a livelihood of sorts for me as long as I wish to continue. As I grow and change, my fans are interested in hearing about it and, if at all possible, seeing it for themselves. The nature of my representation may change but it will continue to be made available to those who desire it.

I see my career going in a direction that befits an older woman and crone-in-training: education, advocacy and sexual mastery. I have become a valuable resource to the community and for those who will come after me. I hope I will always have younger people around me to draw inspiration from and to inspire in return. That exchange of energy and ideas propels the culture forward.

I have had the rare experience of having had significantly more and varied sexual partners than the average person. My training as a health professional, combined with my exhibitionism and feminist perspective, have given me a unique insight into a very complex issue. Some fundamental truths: men are just as sexually oppressed as women, only in different areas; men need tenderness and caring and touching just as much as women (in fact, they are starved for it); women who share their sexuality with kindness as opposed to vindictiveness wield tremendous power; men will follow our rules if we will only articulate them; most men want to see women sexually happy – all they want to do is join in and be a part of the process; men in the grip of sexual arousal and desire are often at their sweetest and most accessible and are easily guided.

I've learned that sexuality is very fluid and that lines blur (especially in the presence of an experienced partner) with little effort. I've come to appreciate the power of sexual arousal and ecstasy to transform people, to heal their spirits, to radically alter their consciousness permanently and for the better. Sexual contact reaches into the depths of a person, transmitting more information in a single moment than can be communicated any other way.

I've learned that the directness of the sexual experience transcends language barriers, that it truly is the international language. Touch is the ultimate and primal universal communication. I've learned that sexual skills can be taught and passed on, like any other skills, for the betterment of the participants.

Currently, bringing women into the sex industry as consumers is very important to me. I want to contribute to a body of work that speaks to their sexuality as opposed to only trying to capture the 'average' male's interest. I want to educate women and empower them to honour their sexuality, for it can save the world. I want to expand the range of sexually explicit material to encompass more varied sexual interests. I want to promote women's control of reproduction. The issue of the dominant culture's attitude toward, and treatment of, my business (and, by extension, sexuality itself), is one I love to address. Taking my sex-positive message to the greater society is very compelling to me now.

EXERCISE: HOW TO RECREATE A PORN MOVIE FANTASY AT HOME

All we do on-screen is play-act the scripts given to us or, if it's an amateur video, the scripts we give ourselves. It's just role-playing around a basic premise or scenario.

First, each of you must pick a character that excites you. Then, you decide what kind of energy you'll be playing with. Next, you'll need to decide on the set-up: where are you supposed to be? You may want to negotiate the type of sex ahead of time, for example, 'rape', 'seduction', 'love fucking', 'sport fucking', a blow job or mutual masturbation.

Then, put on costumes (if you want to) and start playing. Go ahead and play out the role you've chosen. It is the ultimate in improvisational theatre. The idea is to have fun and develop intimacy. If it stops being fun, stop the activity. Keep it up for as long as you feel like it – that's all it takes to make your own porn movie.

9

Women's Sex Shops

In 1962 Beate Uhse opened the first sex shop in the world, the Sex Institute of Marital Hygiene in Flensburg, Germany. She later opened similar shops in other German cities and became a notorious celebrity by doing so. She also set up porn theatres to show what were then known as 'blue' movies – but the market for her adult businesses was most definitely men.

Eve's Garden was the first women's sex shop in the world, established by Dell Williams in 1973. The impetus for it came out of the first Women's Sexuality Conference in New York and from her friendship with Betty Dodson, who was running masturbation workshops for women.

Dell started her business with two mail-order products and ran the business from her home. As the business grew, she developed the product range and in 1978 opened a retail shop on Manhattan's Upper East Side. Her main product lines were books and vibrators, which she hoped would educate women on how to use to have orgasms. This was a major move from the traditional sex shop approach, where there was so much about sexuality still 'unsaid' and the main emphasis was on different lingerie lines to create a sexual atmosphere. Dell was a pro-sex feminist who believed in women's liberation without religious or political interference.

In 1977 Joani Blank opened Good Vibrations in San Francisco which had both a mail-order catalogue service and operated as a shop. It was very different from Xandria and Adam and Eve in San Francisco, the other contemporary mail-order businesses which centred on men's sexual products and needs. The pro-sex environment of Good Vibrations focused on having quality vibrators and videos for women whether they be lesbian, bisexual or heterosexual.

In the early 1990s Hanni Jagtman and Ellen van der Gang set up Mail and Female in Amsterdam, the first mail-order catalogue for women in Europe. They realised that many women were not comfortable in the existing outlets even in liberated Amsterdam. As their business grew they branched out with shops of the same name, and others called Female & Partners in Holland, Belgium and Spain. They found that 80 to 90 per cent of people who contacted them were women, that they were over thirty years of age and looking to purchase vibrators and clothing to improve their sex life.

In Australia in the early 1990s there were still no sex shops designed for women. Sex shops were all based on a male model, typified by rows of 'girlie' magazines and videos, badly designed phallic-shaped vibrators and dildos, and a man (who frequently knew nothing of female sexuality) behind the counter. The overall atmosphere was one of sleaze. For women entering this environment the most common response was frequently embarrassment.

Courses in the area of sex-positive sexuality were already being run and a natural progression was the set-up of The Pleasure Spot in 1992. It was the first mail-order catalogue and later a shop to focus on what women wanted. The design and layout of products in the catalogue were easy for women to purchase from as they included how and why you would use. The main emphasis was on a feminine, sensual, uninhibited, non-sleazy marketing approach. Inspired by goods available in the US new products were designed, which included silicon dildos shaped as whales, dolphins, goddesses and intertwined lovers, plug-in vibrators and videos centring on helpful sex education, female erotica and sensual products. Courses were also available to support women and couples on their sexual journey.

As this was a very different style of business from traditional sex outlets it made competition difficult. The older well-established businesses had large budgets for marketing and advertising while The Pleasure Spot relied on having an upfront media profile for its sex-positive approach. Thousands and thousands of women and their partners responded enthusiastically to this new way of looking at sexuality.

Recently in Japan Minori Kitahara rejected the traditional male Japanese culture she had been brought up in to bravely introduce a new type of sexuality to Japanese women. She followed the trailblazing women in the West through her shop Love Piece and mail-order catalogue.

Ky began Sh! in 1992 in London after being frustrated in her attempts to find basic female sexual products. She felt women's needs were not being addressed in the existing male owned and run shops. The response was fantastic, reflecting what had happened in the US, Holland, Japan and Australia, where women supported other women in this new approach to feminist sexuality.

JO-ANNE BAKER

Putting sexuality in the right perspective

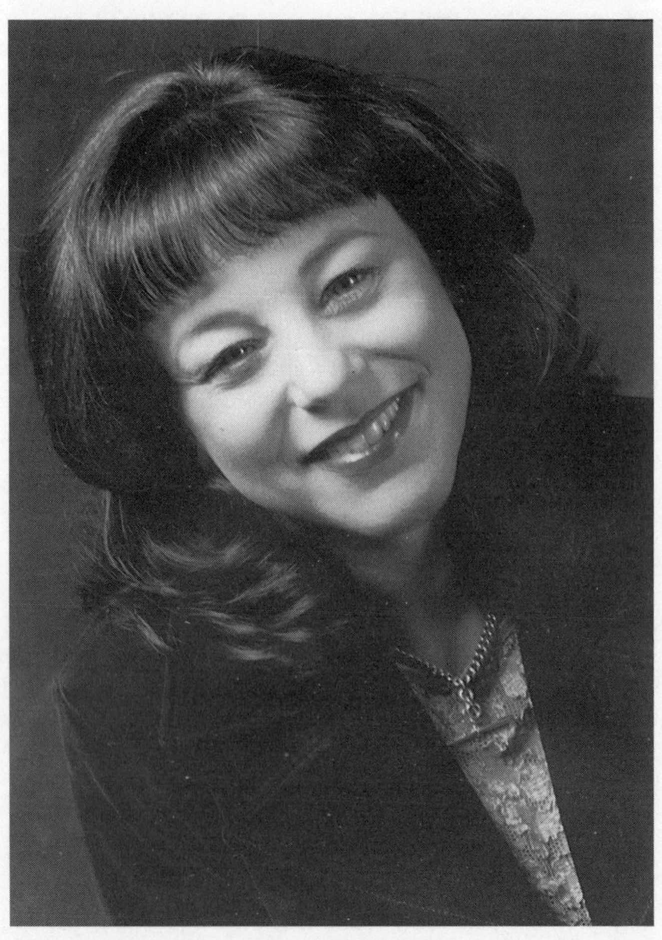

Matthew Scroope

Women's Sex Shops

Jo-Anne Baker has worked in the area of sexuality since 1990. Her business The Pleasure Spot was the first in Australia to focus on women's sexuality and couples. It introduced a wide variety of sex toys, videos and literature which were not previously available, as well as courses on spiritual, sexual growth.

After receiving her sociology degree in Australia Jo-Anne travelled widely and lived in the UK, US and Italy, where she trained in erotic spirituality. This included bio-energetics, hypnotherapy, meditation, Tantra, sex positivism, macrobiotics, astrology and massage. She successfully introduced futons to Australia in the 1980s, revolutionising the bedding market.

She is well-known as one of Australia's leading sex entrepreneurs and educators, and articles about her work have appeared in all national magazines, newspapers, TV and radio. Jo-Anne now focuses on her writing and individual sessions, teaching people to experience more pleasure in their body. Her previous book is Self-sexual Healing.

My quest to understand my own sexuality did not start until the 1980s, when I participated in many self-development courses and workshops that focused on learning how to connect with my body and expand my sensuality. I wanted to heal the sexual repression I had grown up with and learn how to be relaxed with myself.

My journey to find sexual fulfilment took me around the globe, visiting women who have changed history by bringing sexual taboos out of the darkness and teaching women how to experience pleasure, fun and lots of sexual fulfilment. There is never enough time to explore the depth of pleasure and sensuality that could be possible for each one of us.

In 1992 I started The Pleasure Spot, an adjunct to the courses on sexuality I was organising. It was at first a mail-order business and later became the first retail sex shop for women in Australia. I felt it was essential to put sexuality in the right perspective, and remove the connotations that it was dirty, bad or something to be ashamed of. Many sex products and all sex shops had been designed by men, who believed they knew what women wanted, but for many women this was far from true. I visited the existing women's sex shops around the world, including Eve's Garden in New York, Good Vibrations in San Francisco, Sh! in London, Mail & Female in Amsterdam – and all of them inspired me with their innovative approach to sexuality.

When I set up the business I paid special attention to sensual products, such as feathers, candles, edible oils and powders as well as non-phallic dildos. I stocked plug-in vibrators, which were then a novelty in Australia and they quickly caught on.

I sold products and ran and organised courses designed to teach women how to feel more relaxed and alive in their body. The courses included breath and energy orgasms, striptease, erotic massage. They became popular with men too, so I included evenings for couples and men only.

Many women are still embarrassed to visit a sex shop and talk about sexuality because they feel that the area is taboo or they have feelings of shame about their body or their erotic desires. Thousands of women have begun conversations with me at The Pleasure Spot with 'I have never told anyone about this', 'I feel really embarrassed to ask you about this', 'I am probably the only one to feel this way', or 'Is there something wrong with me because I like... I have found that men and women are desperate for clear, accurate sexual information that is free of judgement, sleaze and double entendres.

Overwhelmingly the issues my clients have wanted to discuss haven't surprised me, and I have been able to reassure them that their sexual desires or interests are not only 'normal', but healthy. We live in such a sex-negative culture that any positive information on sexuality and the human body is still desperately sought. It is amazing that since the 1960s we have been able to go to the moon, yet at the turn of the century so many people are still divorced from the body they live in. We all exist because a sexual act created us, and during our life we need to learn to embrace our sexuality to be at emotional and physical peace.

Since 1990 thousands of Australians have contacted me for products and advice. Doctors and therapists have started sending clients to me who had sexual difficulties. This encouraged me to develop my own form of body-orientated sexual-healing sessions and eventually to publish *Self-sexual Healing: Finding Pleasure Within*, a step-by-step guide to healing with practical exercises and techniques.

EXERCISE: THE WAVE

Time: 10-15 minutes
Setting: A room where you will not be disturbed, or in nature
Music: Something sensual, with a repeated melody
Lighting: Natural or candles

I have worked with many people to help them feel more connected to their body. This is a simple exercise to help you relax and expand your physical flexibility. When you feel relaxed with the movement you can take it into lovemaking and masturbation. An added advantage is that it is good for your back!When women give birth their body undulates like a wave. This movement is also reflected in a woman's orgasm – a ripple effect goes through the body. For men this movement helps the pelvis relax in a backwards and forwards motion, rather than the traditional sensations, which are like a band of sexual tension that builds up to ejaculation. The natural sexual movement is exaggerated through the wave exercise. This is deliberate as it teaches you a wonderful way to turn yourself on and pulse the sexual energy throughout the body.

To begin, lie down on the floor with your knees bent. Place your hand on the top of your head and start to move your pelvis backwards and forwards, keeping your lower back on the floor. This is important, otherwise you will put pressure on this part of your back. Initially connect with the sensations as you move your body, becoming conscious of how your head moves. It is very common for people to only feel movement in their pelvis and not their spine or head. Try again, exaggerating the backward and forward motion so that the top of your head and spine start to move.

Allow your inhale to become stronger as if you were breathing through a straw, let the exhale just happen naturally. Incorporate your breath with the movement, on the inhale clench your pelvic floor muscles (which are the muscles you use to stop yourself from urinating) and relax on the exhale. To enable more relaxation to happen you can imagine your pelvis falling, as though into quicksand as you exhale.

As you find your own natural rhythm you can incorporate visualising light moving from your genitals up the body to the top of your head in waves. Let any sound be expressed, especially if you visualise colour or movement in the throat area. You can also incorporate using a vibrator in this exercise. The main focus is on expanding the senses and moving your sexual energy throughout the body and being turned-on.

JOANI BLANK

Talking sex

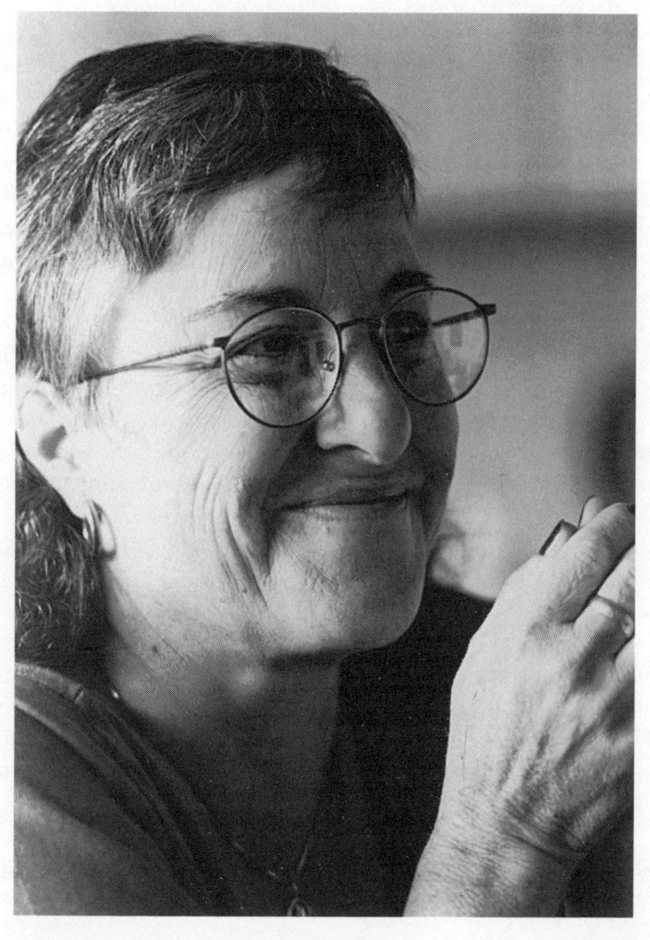

Joani Blank was born in 1937 and raised in Boston. She has a master's degree in Public Health Education with a special interest in family planning, and in the mid-1960s she believed she was headed for a career in international family planning.

When Joani moved to San Francisco in 1971, she realised that sex was a much more intriguing field of inquiry than birth control, although the two fields are apparently related. Joani's realisation that women's difficulties with contraception were connected with their discomfort with their sexuality changed the direction of her life work.

Joani is renowned as the founder of Good Vibrations, San Francisco's famous sex toy, book and video store and mail-order service. Long dedicated to democratic business management, in 1992 she converted Good Vibrations into a worker cooperative; it is now wholly owned by its employees of which she is no longer one.

She also formed Down There Press, Good Vibrations' sister publishing company in 1975, and opened the San Francisco store in 1977. She is author or editor of eight of the fifteen titles currently published by Down There Press. Her books include Good Vibrations, I Am My Lover, A Kid's First Book About Sex, First Person Sexual, Femalia *and the forthcoming* Still Doing It. *In 1996 Joani, doing business as Blank Tapes, produced and directed two videos,* Carol Queen's Great Vibrations *and* Faces of Ecstasy.

Joani has a lot of interests that have nothing to do with sex. One of these is co-housing, a form of cooperative housing that originated in Denmark, and which is spreading with deliberate speed in North America where close to fifty co-housing communities are now built and occupied. She sings in a choir, is learning Taiko drumming, is engaged in socially responsible investing and does volunteer work.

She is a mother and grandmother and would like to be a little less single than she is at present, but she's not quite sure if monogamy works for her.

Dell Williams' business, Eve's Garden, was one of my earliest inspirations. Her business was mail-order but I wanted to open a retail store. My concept was to have a store where people could touch, hold and feel sex toys and be able to have long conversations with staff about the different products.

In 1977 I opened the door to my San Francisco shop, which I called Good Vibrations. My staff are all sex educators and it has always been important to me that they receive very good training.

Good Vibrations has had 150,000 customers, both male and female, since it opened.

What happened during the 1970s in Western society had very little to do with the sexual act itself, but it had to do with the ability of women to control their fertility, via the birth control pill. This basically led to women's liberation. Without this it is unlikely that the women's liberation of the 1970s would have happened with the speed that it did. In terms of the sexual revolution, it is very unlikely that a woman would now grow into adulthood without knowing where her clitoris is and what it is used for. This is very different from when I was growing up.

On some levels things have changed, but in many quarters our society is actually going backwards with regard to sex education as they have Christian-based, abstinence-only sex education programs in schools. These have been proven not to work in terms of preventing STDs and teenage pregnancies. In the process they are creating a generation of kids who, when they do get around to having sex, are going to hate it. Sexual repression is worse because the radical right has created so much negativity about sex. There is now so much more ignorance about sex.

It is my contention that the worst sexual dysfunction we have as a society is our inability to talk about sex. So the thing that interests me the most, and what I like to do in workshops, is to find ways for people to talk about sex. If we could treat sex as just one of a range of things that people do, instead of something special that belongs over there, separate to everything else, we could create a whole different atmosphere around sex. It would be easier to talk about sex, bring it up in conversation and acknowledge a sexual attraction between people.

Instead we have put sex in a place that is separate from the rest of our lives. Sex is not separate from the rest of our lives. I decided recently that psychoanalyst Sigmund Freud was right when he said that at some level everything is about sex. The fact that we put sex aside to make it something special creates an amazing amount of anxiety around all aspects of sexuality. It's problematic because if you say let's get rid of all the anxiety then you get rid of a lot of the excitement too. I do not have a particularly spiritual orientation around sexuality. However, as I get older I can see that the root of our sexual issues – for example, the things that excite us, freak us out, embarrass us and make us anxious – are all reflections of what happens in our everyday life.

I run a variety of sex workshops where I encourage people to communicate more openly. In women's workshops they learn to be more assertive, to show their sexual strength as opposed to weaknesses. To get to the point where she believes that she deserves to receive pleasure, whatever that takes. A woman can learn what she sexually wants through masturbation; she then needs to learn how to honestly convey that to her partner.

In the men's workshops they explore being vulnerable by expressing what they are feeling. In such a workshop a man told me that he had difficulty forming sexual relationships. I told him that the most important thing was to be vulnerable to his partner. He needed to be able to say, 'I have been out on four dates with you, and I am scared to hold your hand'. It is so powerful to say to someone what you are truly experiencing.

I also run a group workshop called How To Get What You Want In Bed Or Wherever Else You Do It. As part of this workshop the group has an open discussion around the various reasons why they have difficulty asserting themselves sexually and asking for what they want. I have found that many people focus on their fear of rejection. In this workshop we face the fear by getting people to ask for what they want and get rejected. We do this with the emphasis on fun and I encourage a lot of laughter. They have to be able to say, 'No, I don't want to'. It's been a very powerful exercise for people because it gets the couples talking about sex.

I did this workshop recently at a Unitarian Church retreat for about fifteen people, made up of couples and singles of all sexual orientations. After the course it opened up the way they started talking about sex, asking one another about the most interesting places they had masturbated. The people doing the workshop found that you can talk about sex and that it is good. You learn about other people and realise that you are not weird, and not a terrible person for doing it.

My message is to do it! Find fun creative ways to get what you want in bed by deciding who initiates sex, who does what when, what kind of games you like to play and use basic assertiveness techniques. Many people can't imagine that there is any way to talk about sex unless they are in bed, which is not the case. It is important to talk about sex at a non-sexual time. You can also write letters to one another about what you like physically, but make sure it is an equal commitment. In many heterosexual relationships it is often the woman who perceives that she is not getting what she wants from her male partner, while men want to 'fix' their female partners. I tell them to focus on changing themselves first. It does not help a woman to feel as if she is a 'patient' who has to be 'cured' of her problem. Very few people get as much sex as they like or the kind of sex they want. There are also many people who have lots of sex but are not sexually satisfied. I am in my sixties and I am more sexually active and positive than I have ever been in my life.

TIP: HOW TO HAVE A BETTER ORGASM

If you are doing all the right things but still having difficulty coming, here's a tip that works well for me. First, decide how aroused you are on a scale from one to ten. Do not change the stimulation, but pay attention to how warm you are, the amount of tension you have in your legs, and what you are experiencing in your body. This includes how genitally turned-on you feel. Then try to intentionally lower the number you have decided on.

For example, if you decide that on the scale your level of arousal is `eight', then try to intentionally bring your level of arousal to a lower level and a lower number without changing the level of stimulation you are giving yourself. Try to make yourself less aroused. This is a paradoxical instruction. When you tell yourself to be less aroused by trying to lower the number on your scale of arousal, the opposite naturally occurs and you become more excited.

KY

Tune into your true erotic nature

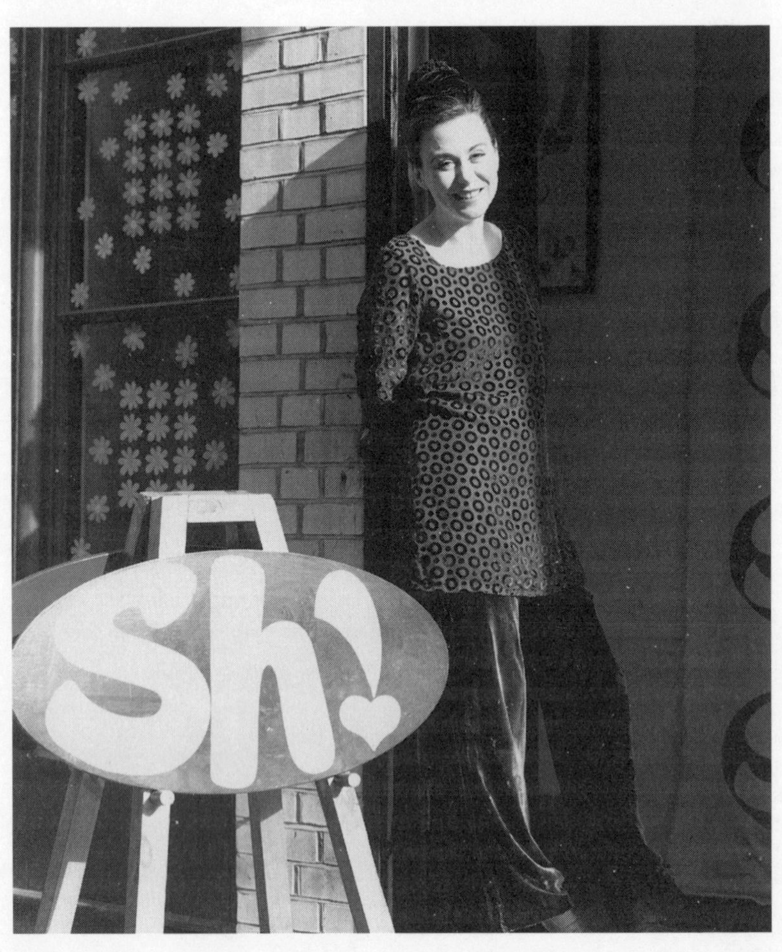

Ky is originally from Yorkshire, UK, and after leaving school, studied at Art School and did a degree in Alternative Practice. In her words, she 'pratted around', including periods being unemployed, stints as a nanny and working in Japan teaching English. She is the proprietor of Sh!, a women's erotic emporium in London.

The inspiration for Sh! started in 1992, when I went shopping with a close friend, Kim, to buy a strap-on dildo and harness for her. We started in Soho and then spread our search to the sex shops around London. We started in inner London and then moved outward in greater concentric circles until it got ridiculous. We went from shop to shop, amazed that we couldn't find what she wanted.

All the dildos and harnesses were either crappy and badly designed, impractical with no idea what a woman wanted or they were made for gay leather men, leather daddies, with all the dildos in realistic penis shapes. At first we thought this was funny, but soon it became depressing and very demoralising.

I found that many sex shops we went into were very uncomfortable when we went in and I got the strong feeling that we weren't supposed to be there. If women often feel uncomfortable in sex shops it is because that is how they are made to feel – as though they are polluting the atmosphere with all their oestrogen, or something. A 1950s atmosphere of 'nice girls don't' pervades many of these shops – and I got really cross about it.

At this time there was a great deal of public sexuality education about AIDS and safe sex and women were urged to talk about what they wanted sexually, the use of condoms and safe sex. I began to wonder what this all meant when women like myself, who considered themselves sexually literate and a sexual outlaws, couldn't find what they wanted. What were straighter, more conservative women going to do? How were they coping?It was during our travels around these sex shops that Kim and I started to discuss opening our own shop for women. It started off as a joke, but as we became more and more annoyed, we became more and more serious about it. Kim was an accountant and she looked into the possibility and thought it was financially feasible. Her encouragement fired me along, but although I was angry at the lack of products for women and believed there was a market for them, I was unsure about whether we could do it.

We went into partnership and opened Sh! in April 1992 with me working in the shop full-time. At first we were so unsure of our own survival we only rented the shop on a week-by-week basis. We started the shop with ?600 and the shop has only ever been in debt once, when we lashed out and bought a company car. The shop has done incredibly well; we have a loyal clientele that travels, often vast distances, to shop with us. We are also fortunate in that we get a lot of media attention.

Our shop is different from sex shop chains supposedly run by women and catering for women. Many of these are a front for straight sex shops that cater mainly to men and use front women as an advertising ploy. We now have two staff, and customer service and care is our number one concern. We have approximately 300 female customers per month, with an even gay-heterosexual split. Plans for the business include deciding whether in the future we want to wholesale our products, the dildos and harnesses we manufacture, and our own handcuffs, collars and other bondage gear.

I believe to have a good sex life you need to learn to tune into your true erotic nature. Come out about what you are interested in without shame. Explore your fantasies and have the courage to live them out, but most importantly ask for what you want sexually.

TIPS ON INTRODUCING SEX TOYS INTO A RELATIONSHIP

- Introduce a sex toy into a relationship either seriously, via a slight power game with bondage or other fantasies, or do it with humour. A note of caution though, if you buy sex toys with a partner be aware that these can become a custody battle in a break-up, so buy your own sexual products.

- Imagination is the key to good sex. I defy anyone not to enjoy at least bondage (with no discipline). It is a wonderful feeling to be strapped down and made love to because you don't have to think about anything - just relax and enjoy the sensations.

• You can sharpen your sexual skills by playing fantasy games - `playing' is the key word. If you can successfully recreate a fantasy character, you can feel that you are having an affair with someone else through the character. I have done this in my own relationship and it has been a lot of fun. Sex toys can give an added dimension to a fantasy game.

• Strap-on dildos for women are the best-selling sex toys at Sh!. It is a very common fantasy for a woman to want to experience wearing a dildo and harness. For a woman to put on a strap-on dildo can be the most embarrassing thing at first, and you can often feel like an idiot. You also don't want your partner to laugh at you! One way to get over this is to blindfold your partner and introduce it that way. This will help you get over your initial awkwardness.

MINORI KITAHARA

Women can orgasm without a penis

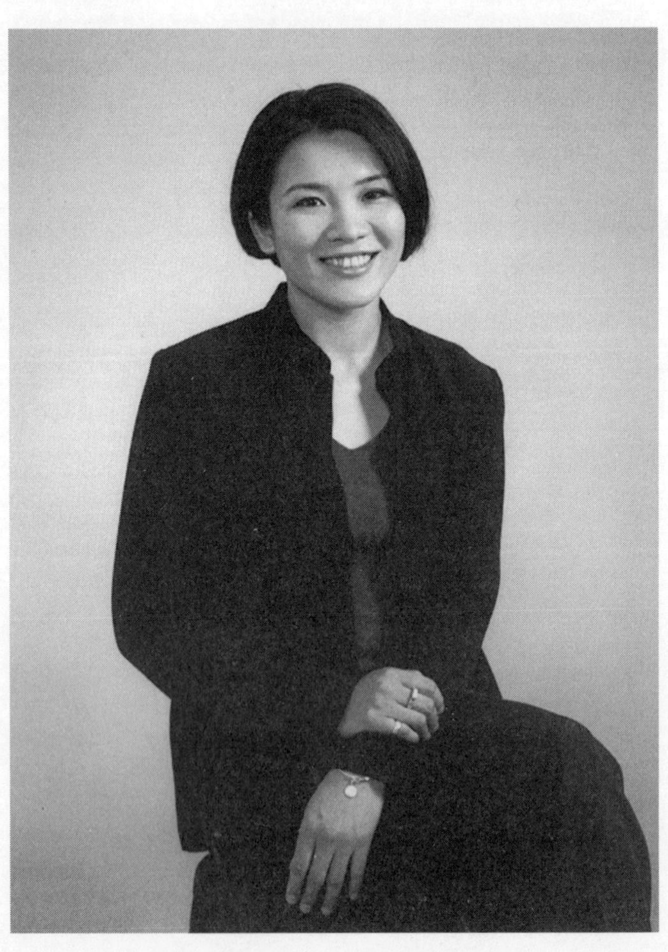

Minori Kitahara was born in Tokyo in 1970 and graduated in the School of Pedagogy at a Japanese tertiary institution. Minori now runs the Love Piece Club, a Tokyo CBD adult shop and design/wholesale warehouse. Minori produces sex educational material for women, including a recent ground-breaking booklet that showed Japanese women how to masturbate. While campaigning for a more open attitude to sexuality in Japan, Minori is also leading the charge to produce non-violent and less overtly macho pornography. In this she is working with Japan's emerging feminist movement.

She has had a long interest in the sex industry. As a young girl she cleaned her grandmother's 'love motel'. Love motels are common throughout Japan, providing a place where couples can go to have sexual privacy as families often live together in relatively small apartments.

When I first read Betty Dodson's book on masturbation, *Self Loving*, I was very moved. I said to myself 'I want to be a Japanese Betty Dodson'. Now, my business is making and selling sex products for women. While we have many sex toys and videos in Japan, almost all of these show the fantasy of men with big penises conquering women. I hate this. Women need to have their fantasies reflected, not just more of the same old porn.

Japan has 12,000 adult shops, about four times the concentration of shops-to-people in Australia, and although non-violent sexually explicit videos are illegal, explicit and savage sexual violence is quite acceptable on film and in print. Dildos and vibrators are also illegal, although if they have a 'face' they are classified as 'dolls' and so are acceptable. This has given rise to the distinctive Japanese vibrator with a woman's or animal's face. To me selling vibrators means freeing women from sex with men.

Prostitution is also illegal, but if a sex worker carries a whip they are safe as they can masquerade as a bondage mistress. It goes without saying that Japan's sex industry and its sexual cultures are confusing.

I have designed and manufactured many innovative products including a disposable dildo made from seaweed gelatine that dissolves in hot water after use. It is ideal for the busy couple who does not wish to leave the 'evidence' in the local love motel, or in their parents' living room.

I have also designed a remote control vibrator/dildo for women.

The woman simply inserts a small projecting section of the sex toy into herself and positions the clit-tickling part, with the aid of snug underwear, before she goes out. While sitting at dinner, working out or on the dance floor or attending church, the vibrator/dildo is activated at will by her partner via a small remote switch. The only problem arises when more than one woman in a room is wearing the sex toy!For women to know what an orgasm is and what is pleasurable for them is very important. When we know this, we love our body more. Masturbation is the easier way to learn this. We can then communicate this to our partner and be open to hearing what turns our partner on.

I don't remember when I started to masturbate, but since I was seven years old I've touched my genitals every night in bed before sleeping in order to feel comfortable. I remember my first orgasm – it was very sensational and happened when I was thirteen. One day I took a shower as usual, but the water pressure on my genitals gave me my first orgasm. Many of the women who come to my shop talk about having their first orgasm in this way and often they can come during masturbation but not during sex.

It is not important to me to have an orgasm during sex, because for me sex is just a communication with people I love. In short, orgasm is not the purpose of sex. But many men are very afraid that women can orgasm without a penis. And many women still feel guilty that they have an orgasm by masturbation.

10

Women with Women

When women are surveyed about their sexual fantasies the fantasy of making love with another woman is always high on the list. The fantasy of breast touching breast, another soft body like their own pressed against them and feeling genitals with a sexual rhythm like their own seems to occupy many women's sexual imagination. The question is not `why a woman would be attracted to another woman' but why wouldn't she? A woman can offer someone of her same sex a great deal in an intimate loving relationship. To women, another woman's particular emotional needs are not seen as peculiar or `other', but innately normal.

A woman knows how the female body works, and has a first-hand insight into the nature of women's erotic pleasure. Women also have more sexual staying power, with the ability to have multiple orgasms and make love for hours on end. Put two of them in a bed together and you have dynamite.

When people are asked to place themselves on Alfred Kinsey's scale of 1-10, in which each end represents either absolute heterosexuality or absolute homosexuality, few people see themselves as immovably at either end. Most people recognise that there is an ambiguity about their sexuality and given the right time, place or circumstance, an experience of loving someone of the same sex is quite possible. However, there is a gender difference here. Overwhelmingly more women than men admit being open to the possibility of loving another woman.

Many women are naturally bisexual, but feel constrained by societal mores in the expression of that sexuality. For others suddenly feeling sexually attracted to, or falling in love with, another woman comes out of the blue and can be a life-changing experience. Lesbianism - despite being the subject of endless straight erotic films - is still more taboo than gay male homosexuality and surveys show that it is less socially acceptable. Every woman who decides to love another woman has to face a number of issues - negotiating a very different kind of sexuality, possibly `coming out' to friends and family, and learning to love and live in a very different manner.

Later in this chapter the contributors to this book who have had erotic interludes with other women offer their insights, experiences and tips in this area. One woman who has written on this is American sexuality author Susie Bright, and here she gives a practical and witty introduction to the concept of a woman picking up another woman.

SUSIE BRIGHT

Lesbians and straight men have a lot in common

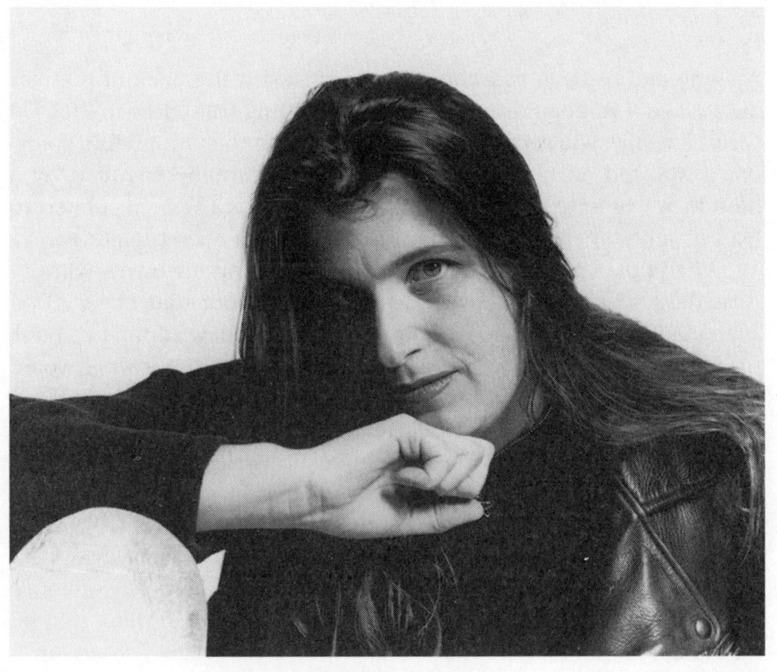

Jill Posener

Susie Bright is known as an editor, notorious sexual activist, advocate of sexual liberation and performer. She is the author of Susie Bright's Sexual Reality, Susie Bright's Lesbian Sex World, Sexwise *and her best-seller,* The Sexual State of the Union. *She is editor of the 'Herotica' series of books and* Best American Erotica.

Susie co-founded On Our Backs, *and served as editor for six years. In 1981 she began working at Good Vibrations, San Francisco's one-of-a-kind vibrator and sex toy shop, where she created the first progressive feminist erotic video library. She lives in San Francisco and has a seven-year-old daughter.*

The following material is extracted from Susie Bright's article, 'How to Make Love to a Woman: Hands on Advice From a Woman Who Does' (originally printed in Esquire magazine).

As long as I've been searching for promises in the back of popular magazines, I've been drawn to that captivating title 'How to Pick Up Girls'. I'm sure you recall the ad. In addition to the untoppable come-on, it showed an average-looking bachelor carnally engulfed by a blonde, a brunette and a redhead. His little smirk was calculated to lead us all to speculate on what his magnificent secret might be.

When I became old enough to pick up girls on my own – without a single guidebook to assist me – I thought about that cheesy Don Juan and whether I had acquired for free the wisdom his book promised for $19.95. Sometimes, during nights on the town, I would catch men staring at me and my latest girlfriend, their looks a combination of envy, bewilderment and titillation. Their eyes seemed to beg for an answer to the question, 'How?'.

Lesbians and straight men do have a lot in common. Both are hung up on girls. We vie for the same joy. It's only natural for each of us to wonder if the other is having more success at it. Lesbians are certainly outmanoeuvred by straight men – in numbers, influence and earning power. And they have penises. But I often think that if I had one, I'd really know what to do with it. (And I don't mean cut it off.) Lesbians know female sexuality from both sides, and so we have an internal, almost incestuous intimacy with the subject. It gives us a wisdom that can't be measured.

But it can be shared.

Suppose, for example, that I wrote a book called 'How to Pick Up Girls Using the Real Live Dyke Method', including informative chapters on the following subjects.

The Look

For most humans, attraction begins with seeing. Look at her. All over. Linger anywhere you like. When she notices (and she will if you're really looking), hold her eyes with yours – hold them close. Every second will feel like a minute. This is the essence of cruising, and it is the experience that virtual reality and phone sex will never replace. It is also the one moment of truth: you'll know then and there whether she wants you or not. If she does want you, she'll be thrilled by your look, because it says to her that she has your full attention.

If she doesn't want you, she'll complain to her friends about how you 'objectified' and 'degraded' her, but ignore all that crap. Calling a man a sexist interloper is just a trendy way of stating an old-fashioned sentiment 'He's not my type'. When a dyke gets an unwanted ogling from another dyke, we don't use political pejoratives. We just say, 'Over my dead body'. Don't confuse looking with watching. 'Girl-watchers' check out every passing femme; to look, as Webster so gracefully defines it, is 'to exercise the power of vision'.

The Touch

Lesbians, too, have probing, yearning, insistent sex organs. We call them hands. And if you have not had the pleasure of taking a woman in your hands – your thumb parting her mouth, your fingers tracing her ears, your hand curled up inside her – you are missing some of the finer points of ecstasy. Use your hands like they're your tenderest parts. The sweetest confession I ever made to a man was this: 'You use your hands like a dyke.' Lesbians often say that making love to a woman feels right because 'It's like touching yourself'. It's a flimsy reason for choosing a partner, but a good general motto for any lover. Touch your lover the way you would touch yourself. It's about empathy, not road maps. Every part of her corresponds to a part of you.

The Surrender

Consensual rough stuff aside, the thought that emotionally mature women (meaning no nut cases) enjoy mean and nasty treatment is way outta line. Women are invariably turned on by men who can be tender – it's like watching a statue cry, very moving. A woman hopes she will see more of this, and so she perseveres. Most times she learns that he's only vulnerable three days out of the year, and it's not worth the other 362 to wait for the High Holy Days.

Personality-wise, you either have that candour and softness to express or you don't, but sexually, anyone can lie back once in a while. Not every girl wants to get in the saddle and grab the reins, but if you have the slightest inkling that your woman would like to run this fuck, say a silent prayer and let her do whatever she wants.

My book would offer all that and more. But remember this bit of final wisdom: picking up girls is the easiest part of love. When it comes to seduction, you can try a dozen successful techniques. It's holding onto affection and lust that remains unteachable. The beginning of love is only the promise of all that's to come – for boys and for girls. Remember, it all begins with a look, which is nothing more than a hope, and if I can seduce a straight girl with the strength of my curious green eyes, then you shouldn't have any problem at all.

Annie Sprinkle: For any woman who wants to explore herself sexually with another woman, find a woman who defines herself as a lesbian, or who has had other female lovers. Avoid going after a heterosexual woman because there is a high possibility of rejection. I have seen some women frustrated and hurt by this mistake.

Shelly Mars: Ask friends who they know are lesbians to set you up with someone. Lesbian bars are not my first choice. It is not that much different than a heterosexual relationship – while courting you go out to dinner, and if they drink, get some wine and go home. I think a massage is always the best way to break the ice, because it relaxes someone. You can have a conversation while doing it, and it's sensual but non-threatening.

If you feel that there is chemistry, kiss the other person and go from there. Foreplay is no different whether you are with a man or a woman. If you are a woman you have a woman's body, so you automatically know what feels good and you have an advantage over men. If appropriate you could use some sex toys, and ask her if it feels good.

Diane Torr: Hmm. I have a game that I play which goes like this:I do something you want for x amount of time, such as massage back, suck toes, stroke hair.

You do something I want for x amount of time, such as kiss me all over my body, paddle my buttocks, lick me behind the knees.

I do something you want... and so on. This is GUARANTEED to break the ice and is also a lot of fun.

norrie mAy-welby: My tip is to make sure you're the same species as her. Any human is capable of sexually fulfilling any other. If you're used to playing fixed gender roles, it may be useful to let these go. If everyone's waiting for someone else to be 'the man', nothing is gonna happen.

The first time I ended up in bed as a woman with another woman, I remembered that my lesbian friends complained about straight women who laid back and expected the lesbian to do all the work. I resolved I wasn't going to be like that, because I identified as being good in bed! So, I did my fair share of giving and receiving, and was flexible about who took what roles.

Be responsive to your partner. Don't be afraid to do things that you may never have done with a man. Allow yourself to receive pleasure as well as give it. Penetration may or may not be part of what you, or she, wants. Don't assume it is, and don't assume it isn't. There is no set of orgasm techniques. Every woman is different, and may even change herself from moment to moment.

Let go of expectations and preconceptions. Be as present in the moment as possible, and be with what's actually happening, not what you think 'should' be happening. Respect stated and unspoken boundaries. You both have a right to say 'yes, there, more', or 'no, not there', and change your mind at any moment. Most of all, bring your sense of humour to bed with you, and let yourself laugh, cry or moan as the mood takes you.

Carol Queen: Ask her what she likes and do your best to give it to her! If she's not sure or can't say, do lots of things and have her give you feedback about what she prefers. Or give her erotic stories or videos to read or watch and find the parts she likes and wants to try.

In general (though there are exceptions), women like body contact. Our entire skins can be erogenous zones, so a lighter touch moving to more forceful or stronger touch as arousal builds; a wet, not dry, clitoris; and many women love clitoral stimulation along with vaginal or anal thrusting – again, wet, so have lubricant handy!These physical tendencies say nothing of the emotional ones (does she like to be aggressive or be taken? does she want sex within a context of love and commitment? or does she like to be out on the prowl?). Each woman is different and anyone wanting to please a particular woman has to pay attention to her responses and expressed desires.

Kimberly O'Sullivan: You haven't lived until you have loved another woman.

Ruth Ostrow: My only comment to anyone wanting to experiment is go for it!

Cleo Dubois: I come from a predominantly heterosexual background. When I came out into the scene in the very early 1980s it was the beginning of many self discoveries. I explored some simple kinky activities with women – spanking or whipping, for instance. In the queer community that welcomed me some women were interested in playing with me as a submissive.

With them, and also with some gay leathermen, I discovered the joys of getting vaginally fisted. What an incredible, ecstatic, transformative experience! Until then I had no idea this practice even existed! For me it created a link between big orgasmic space, profound emotional depth and spiritual awakening. From there, I began to identify as bi-kinky, playing often with non-separatist leatherdykes as well as non-separatist gay leathermen. Now, I certainly feel comfortable identifying as bisexual, although I'm not as confident of my sexual talents with another woman as I'd like to be.

Aggressive leatherdykes are the ones, and I hope will continue to be the ones, who have initiated with me if they are interested in play. I haven't had much experience with or much desire to be the initiator with femme kinky lesbians. There isn't a quick fix for these – for sex between women to happen at least one of them has to have some aggressive desires, and then I can't be guaranteed that I'll get 'done' back! The ideal would be that both of you want each other, and are vying for top or aggressive space. You'll just have to take turns! It's hard for me sometimes, when women flirt with me, and then won't do anything about it. I realise that they want me to do them, but if I'm not too interested, it just won't work.

I wish that we had the simplicity and directness that gay men have when cruising, picking each other up, and making things happen. I'm looking forward to reading others' stories in this book to find some tips on how to do that! Gay men are also great at communicating their needs, 'Rub this way, no that way, more there, do this, do that.' Women seem to find articulating their needs that way very hard.

My friend Annie Sprinkle has created a fabulous workshop on Ecstatic Yoni Massage involving all kinds of techniques of pussy arousal, as well as anal awakening to pleasure workshop, which I always recommend for men and women whenever it is offered. If you get a chance to attend, go for it. For women being sexual often seems to involve something of the heart. Gay men are so clear about sex for its own sake. We women are so much more complex!In my work with couples I have been happy to help women with no real same-sex experiences. Again it seems that the mixture of role-play and sensuality can open some doors that had been kept locked, although the fantasy has been there for a long time. That is a joy!

Kat Sunlove: As a bisexual, I have always found women desirable. As an assertive woman, I have rarely had trouble expressing that desire. My first experience with a woman is perhaps illustrative. My lover at the time was a handsome black man who knew of my interest in women. We were entertaining Jane, a close friend of mine from college, for the weekend. She and I had teased sexually over the years and had virtually traded boyfriends in school, but we had never acted on our erotic thoughts for one another. When Kenneth confided to me his desire for my friend, it excited me so much that I decided to try to make something happen.

When Jane prepared for a shower, I asked if I might join her and wash her back. The electricity between us at that moment told me all I needed to know. Had her reaction not been so clear, I'm not sure that we would have ended up in bed as we did. A simple opening like that is not as difficult as a full-fledged seduction, persuading a reluctant female to explore the unknown that way.

But just as with SM, following the energy is the safest way I know to explore sexual territory. If you feel an erotic charge when you look in a woman's eyes or touch her hand by accident, you should feel fairly confident that, if she is at all self-aware, she too is feeling the same thrill. Whether or not she would wish to act on that impulse is the risky part. Be brave. Look at her with intent in your eyes. Let her see your desire and if desire answers back, you will probably know what to do next.

Dolores French: I think being really direct is important and meeting women at events or places where there are lesbians or bisexuals. When you meet someone you are attracted to and you are interested in experimenting with them, let them know and be direct. If you don't have the guts you won't have the glory!

Nina Hartley: First, educate yourself about the nature of female sexuality, anatomy and biology. A woman is drawn to confidence, people who are at home in their skin and can transmit that to her. A woman is drawn to people who are comfortable with touching: learn to receive and give massage. Learn to kiss and pet. Learn to love cats (if you don't already). Develop control over your own desire and arousal. Be patient in bringing her up to your level. Don't be a user.

Learn to cook a couple of things: breakfast and a late-night snack. Show consideration. Learn to appreciate beauty and art. Being able to dance helps get a woman in a receptive mood. Learning emotional literacy and being able to communicate effectively is of tremendous assistance. To fulfil a woman, you must arouse her desire, make her want to be naked with you. The above-mentioned skills are most useful in this task.

It helps to choose a sex partner who already masturbates, who knows her body and can tell you what pleases her. To fulfil a woman takes willingness and the ability to tune into her, to honour her desires, even when they don't mesh with yours. Try, to the best of your abilities, to help her live out her fantasies without disrespecting yourself in the process. If a woman feels safe, respected and beautiful, she will be the most wonderful partner you can imagine.

Nan Kinney: To heterosexual women who want to explore their

sexuality with other women I say good sex is all about communication. Communicating your desires to your partner whether you're straight, gay, bi or whatever. There's no one way to fulfil everyone. You have to find out what your potential partner wants by whatever way you're good at: romance, reading a book together, playfulness, pretend, dress-up, watching a movie (any kind of movie; a porn movie would be best) together. Do whatever you can to open communication, to get the talking or writing going.

If you don't have a potential partner, try a workshop or read a book. Kim Airs at Grand Opening, a women's sexuality shop in Boston, does a very successful workshop for women who want to explore lesbianism. Or you can read something like Virgin Territories about first times for women. See what's on the shelves in your local book shop.

Should you go to a lesbian bar? Not with your boyfriend, not if you want a real lesbian! But seriously, if you're comfortable in bars, try it. See how you feel in a lesbian bar. Notice the women you're attracted to. Make eye contact. See if they return the contact. Then start a conversation. Talk about anything – baseball, politics, traffic. Bring a book or magazine with you and mention an interesting article or author you're reading. Buy her a drink. Words of advice, though: don't ever seduce a drunk woman. I don't believe drunk women can make cognitive choices about having sex. But you can get her phone number and meet for dinner or lunch at another time.

If you're not comfortable in bars, try lesbian events such as a reading at your local book shop, or a softball game, or a motorcycle convention! Or church. Do everything the same minus the drinks. Just remember to be yourself and not somebody you're not. Don't put on some image of 'lesbian' for lesbians. When you're comfortable with yourself you are at your most attractive to other people. Relax. And if it doesn't happen the first time, there's always tomorrow. And there's always the vibrator when you go home.

Jo-Anne Baker: Communication is the key. If you are interested in someone, telling them that you are attracted to them will either take the connection further or clearly show you there is no interest. Why spend days, weeks or months worrying whether someone likes you? It is so liberating to be able to just say it!In the traditional male-female roles, there is much game-playing. Women are meant to wait until a man shows interest, phones, asks you out, then you wait again for him to contact you, if at all. If you ring a man you are considered too pushy, too easy, too strong. In relationships with a woman the power dynamic is more equal. Unless same-sex couples rely on gender stereotyping by taking on traditional male-female roles.

Ky: Being with a man is more problematic than being with another woman!

11

Celibacy

Asking about celibacy in the hypersexual late 1990s is like asking someone their financial status, religion or political leaning – it is not deemed a suitable topic for conversation. Many women feel ambivalent about celibacy – is it a choice, a curse, a failure, a period of closed-off meditation or a new way to view the world? Some women feel constrained by its solitariness, others freed by it. The question seems to hinge on whether women felt it was chosen or externally imposed.

Many people are confused about whether celibacy means refraining from sexual activity at all, or only sexual activity with another, meaning that masturbation is okay. Here we have taken celibacy to mean being sexually with yourself, not with another.

For many single people going without sex for weeks, months or even years is not uncommon, yet the perception persists that this represents some kind of sexual failure. Celibacy is frequently portrayed as the refuge of the desperate, dateless, old and unappealing. But is celibacy chosen because of a lack of available sexual partners or a lack of suitable ones? Many women choose celibacy to break destructive sexual patterns from repeating themselves. Others choose celibacy when they are in a state of sexual change or development, and some women when they do not want the distraction of a lover because they want to focus on their own creative growth.

Celibacy is not related to age, yet there is a wide-held belief that the older you become the less sex you have, so that by the time you reach your sixties, seventies or eighties then celibacy is inevitable. For those celibate in their twenties or thirties this view is very destructive and people can falsely believe that if they are not sexual during this time, they will never have sex again.

There seems to be a stigma in our society that if you are in a relationship you should be having sex as often as possible. To be celibate but involved with someone is considered to be even worse than being single and celibate. In such a situation many people believe that there must be something 'wrong' between the partners. While there may be sexual issues that need to be addressed, many couples go through periods of celibacy without the love and commitment between them suffering in any way. Many people in long-term successful partnerships find other ways to show intimacy rather than have sex. If both are content with this situation it must be accepted as a valuable way of loving.

Asking about celibacy proved to be one of the most controversial questions in this book, even to women working in the area of sexuality. Frequently it elicited a surprised silence, embarrassment or even defensiveness from women who were otherwise articulate and sexually confident.

Annie Sprinkle: Sometimes celibacy can be a really positive experience. I have talked to many women whose celibate phases have formed an important part of their sexual evolutions. I know some people make the commitment not to have sex for an entire year or for a month because they wish to devote that sex time and energy to a specific project or heal from an ended relationship. I have even known people who have had long sexual relationships with a partner and decided that they were going to, within that relationship, take a year not to be sexual together. It can be like an intermission from the passion and drama. Then you come back together totally renewed and rekindled. There is a fine line between healthy celibacy and sexual repression, so be careful. Try to be clear about why you are choosing celibacy, whether you are happy about it or not. If you are not, change it. You can try to repress your sexuality, but it is going to be there, it will never go away. You might be able to sublimate it temporarily, but the sleeping dragons will awake and you will have to deal with them.

I don't know anyone who is celibate who does not masturbate. As far as I know, everyone on the planet masturbates – as Dr Jocelyn Elders says, '90 per cent of all people masturbate, and the other 10 per cent lie about it'.

Elizabeth Burton: I think celibacy can be a positive thing because you can have time for yourself and can spend it getting to know who you are. There have been times when I rushed into going to bed with someone just for the sake of sex and felt sad and unfulfilled afterwards; I felt I had let myself down. If you are not in a fulfilling relationship then you are either celibate or in and out of relationships. I don't want to be in and out of relationships – I would rather wait until the right person comes along.

Linda Montano: Celibacy can be a wonderful prayer.

Cora Emens: There might be a time for celibacy in everybody's life.

Even though I never thought it would happen to me, since I absolutely enjoy sex, it did. Why? Because it did not feel right to have sex. There was no real longing for sharing since I was so busy getting to know myself on a spiritual plane. That was very important to me then so I basically declared myself a 'virgin' again, thus reclaiming full responsibility over my sexuality and my body. What I did from that point on was totally up to me.

During my spiritual quest I definitely found something to work with and to work for. It is as if I understood my purpose in life. And that was the end of my celibacy! I am still very happy with myself and that I took the time to reflect on myself instead of indulging in the ever-more meaningless pursuit of sex. Instead of renouncing my virginity, however, I announced my femininity.

Now I have a life partner and we both enjoy a free and sexually open lifestyle with a nice mixture of meaningful and meaningless sex (!) and are helping to liberate others through the media. I believe that celibacy can be a good thing to experience, but we must understand that it comes for all persons in their own time, and we can never force 'morality' on people – in the end they will behave how and with whom they choose no matter what.

Jwala: This is something I don't know much about. I have always wanted lovers and had them in my life. The longest I have gone without a lover my adult life is five weeks and the second longest was four weeks. Both times I had finished a relationship and was in a mourning process. When I finished mourning I met someone new to be sexual with. I express myself sensually and kinesthetically so lovemaking and a love affair have been important for me.

Kutira: True celibacy is not a denial or suppression of sexual energy. It is when one chooses to focus or channel sexual energy in non-sexual ways into life itself. There are times in our lives when this can be a personal love affair with oneself, and an important phase in becoming ready to be in a healthy loving relationship.

Diane Torr: This can be a time when you see no opportunity for sexual fulfilment in your life. It could be self-imposed in that you are 100 per cent focused on a project, and don't want to be distracted in any way. It could also be a time in your life that you want to figure some things out. In a positive way, I think of celibacy as akin to fasting. You're cleaning the slate so that you can have a chance to recuperate, and centre yourself and learn about your sexual needs by focusing inwards. However, can you still be considered celibate if you masturbate? In my own experience, celibacy hasn't always been satisfying or self-imposed. I'm just coming out of a relationship where there was a sexual drought for a number of years. It feels great to be horny and I know I can reasonably expect sexual fulfilment with my new partner. What a relief!

norrie mAy-welby: I have never consciously chosen celibacy, and have often felt frustrated when experiencing long periods of abstinence. Sometimes I could see these periods were a result of my lifting my expectations (through improving my own self-esteem), and finding that the available suitors would not be likely to meet my new personal standards. I have also had long periods without relationships where I was radically exploring myself in ways that I may not have if I was worried about my partner's reactions.

I have tried to ease my frustration in celibacy by making lists of what needs I have met from a relationship, and then finding alternative means of meeting those needs. I try to maintain a healthy sexual relationship with myself, and not be completely dependent on someone else to fulfil my sexual needs.

Shelly Mars: I did have a period over a year when I was celibate and I think that celibacy is a very healing time, where you go into yourself completely and fully. It's interesting when the sexual drive goes away and you are just with yourself and you become all right about it. I think you focus in more on yourself when you are celibate.

If people are in a relationship and celibate, I would at first think they were having some problems they need to work out. However, as I get older, I realise relationships fit everyone's needs, and if they are happy to be celibate and don't care, why should I?

Carol Queen: I have not actually been celibate by choice – that is, I have not made a conscious decision to refrain from sex with others, which is how I mainly understand the term. However, I have been celibate for periods of time (a year and longer) in my adult life, because I haven't had a partner and haven't chosen to look for another; also, I have been celibate for stretches of a few months while with partners with whom I wasn't being sexual, usually because the relationship was somehow in disarray.

Sometimes this 'non-consensual celibacy' has actually been exactly what I needed, especially as it has been a grounding force that brought me back to myself when I was too focused on someone else.

I have not undergone any great length of celibacy in which I've refrained from masturbation, and I do not see that I would ever choose to do this. However, at different times I have more or less sexual energy, so sometimes I go for periods of time without masturbating – but never by design. It simply has to do with my energy levels.

Kimberly O'Sullivan: I was always very relationship-dependent, starting my first long relationship, of six years, when I was only thirteen. In retrospect it was way too young. I subsequently spent my entire sexually active adult life, until recently, in relationships or being actively promiscuous between them. I had absolutely no idea what it was like to sleep alone, or to not have a sexual partner.

When at forty-one I became abruptly single, and non-consensually celibate, I raged in fury against the universe. I felt in a state of utter abandonment, I had no frame of reference to see myself as an independent, sexually whole, single woman. I spent the next twelve months doing sexual therapy and counselling, exploring my own sexuality, meditating and going within to search for answers.

I wanted to reconstruct my life, and was determined not to repeat the same old mistakes I had made. When I came to the realisation that there was no way I could do this without being single and celibate, I came to see my sexual and emotional state as a gift, not a punishment.

I now look at my year of celibacy as the best thing that could have happened to me sexually and emotionally. When I started having (plenty of) sex again I realised that something deep had shifted, I felt free of the desperate compulsion to be coupled – and my fear of aloneness had disappeared.

Ruth Ostrow: I have had long periods of time without a partner during my life but I have never considered myself celibate because I have had such fabulous fun making love to myself! In fact, some of my best orgasms ever have been at my own hand.

Rosie King: In many cultures and societies celibacy is very much valued. We are living in a particularly sexually obsessed era, where we practise 'musterbation' (not masturbation, which is good for us). 'Musterbation' is the belief that everyone must be having sex, but every need you get out of sex can be met in other ways. You can express love and affection in non-sexual ways, you can have physical fun and pleasure in sport or other activities. You can experience a feeling of passion in work, community or family. Anything that delights the senses will fulfil sensual needs, such as having a warm bath, playing beautiful music, applying lovely oils to your skin, massaging your feet, having a facial or just brushing your hair.

To deal with the need for skin hunger you can use appropriate means of touch and affection, by playing with animals or with children. Studies of dogs used in nursing homes and hospitals have shown that contact with pets seems to have a healing power, and the patient's health improves. All our sexual needs, including sexual release, can be met without sexual contact with another. Much worse than not having a sexual partner or regular sex is having sex with someone you don't like.

Many people are involuntarily celibate, which feels very painful if it has been forced upon you. Alex Comfort, who wrote the *Joy of Sex*, said that old people give up sex for the same reasons people give up riding a bicycle – because they are not fit enough, because they think it looks silly or they don't have a bicycle. There are many women out there who don't have bicycles. The Australian woman can expect, on average, up to ten years of widowhood, so we are left with an increasing population of older women without partners. Sexual fulfilment through solo sexual activity is something that women need to explore, because you can have a terrific sex life on your own.

Tuppy Owens: I have used periods without shared sex to discover new sexual responses, but I hate the idea of not sharing a bed, if not every night, with someone I love and fancy. I also think that every day seems grey when there's not one possibility that you might have a sexual encounter. I know there are Tantric practices that involve abstaining for months, with a fantastic outcome, but I can't see myself having the patience. I have always found that the more sex you have, the better it becomes.

Amanda Dwyer: I think celibacy is unnatural. If celibacy is self-inflicted I believe it would be because that person has no sex drive whatsoever, or has taken an oath or vow for religious or spiritual purposes. If one finds oneself celibate because of circumstances within a relationship where one partner shows no interest, I think celibacy then becomes an imposed sentence.

Many of my personal clients have wives who are fully aware of their relationship and visitations with me and my establishment. Obviously, many people eventually make a decision. They come to a point where they either seek out a partner purely for sexual gratification, or they live in hope of things somehow magically changing within their personal relationship. I would see that decision as based on the level of commitment and trust that exists within the relationship. As long as commitment and trust are involved there is always room for growth and the ability to overcome most negative things.

Cleo Dubois: First of all, I have to ask what do we mean by 'celibacy'? I once asked a female Episcopalian priest who came to me for a bondage and spanking session what she meant when she told me she was celibate. She said: 'I do not have a vow, and of course I masturbate!' Does it mean being out of touch with your sexuality for a while, experiencing a lack of sexual drive because of loss, grief, depression, relationship difficulties, health problems or hormonal life changes, even out of a positive choice?I have a usually very sexually active woman friend who chose, after a relationship ended, to remain celibate for a year, except for masturbation, just to see how it would be. Obviously there's a big difference between chosen celibacy and having either no desire or wanting, but not having, a partner to have sex with.

During the mid-1970s I travelled to Guam, where there is a large American military base, and for six months was isolated and without company. I didn't to want to pick up sailors in bars, and only had sex with my vibrator. That's how I discovered I was multi-orgasmic! At another time in my life, I was very depressed, and although I was married, and had a community of possible play partners, I didn't feel like sex at all. It was only when I sorted out my issues through therapy that my sex drive came back.

So my experience of celibacy has been limited, but both positive and negative. I have read, and heard from women friends, though, that a period of celibacy can be empowering and centring, a time to find out how central your sexuality is to your identity.

Another friend was unpartnered for a while and non-consensually celibate. Having tired of her vibrator, she turned to the Internet and started to have lots of cybersex. In the process she tells me she found out a great deal about the nature of her desires and her fantasy life, which she subsequently brought into her real-life relationship when one eventually came along.

In my work with couples who are discovering the joys and challenges of BD/SM, it is not rare that the woman confides in me that the excitement of the new possibilities of role-playing brings sexual desire back into her life – and in a way where her whole body and mind become part of the arousal.

Kat Sunlove: Well, there's celibacy and then there's orgasmic retention. Layne, my husband, and I practised the latter in our early explorations of SM, deliberately allowing the Kundalini energy to build up to boiling point. It can be breath-taking when you are finally allowed to come. Orgasmic retention can make you want sexual contact so much that you are willing to do almost anything just for the mystery sensation you crave. The senses are heightened by deprivation. That alone is an argument in favour of celibacy.

In later years, as we found ourselves less satisfied by routine SM play, Layne and I floundered around in our relationship, looking for an erotic combination that met both of our needs. We wanted to be sexual with one another because we were, and still are, very much in love. But the spectacular sexual experiences that we had enjoyed were not forthcoming with straight sex. We experimented with other people, as we always had in our very open relationship, and had some fun outside our primary partnership. But eventually we agreed that we would not work at sex, but rather would simply love one another and allow the sex to be there or not, without judging our relationship in a negative way if we chose not to be physical in our affection.

Currently, we are physically intimate very infrequently, either together or with others, but neither of us seems to mind. We love one another and know that we have enjoyed years and years of some of the best sex anyone could ever hope to have! And we fully expect we will again.

Deborah Sundahl: Celibacy often signals a time of change in one's sexuality, one's desires or orientation or style. The old you is giving way to a new you, as yet unnamed and unformed, and so a transition period is necessary. And celibacy – refraining from regular sexual activity – emerges. Sometimes this is a death of the libido altogether, and sometimes it is a choice to retain and acknowledge the erotic impulse, but not to satisfy it at all, or in the usual way by engaging in masturbation or partnered sex.

Celibacy is normally a temporary state, lasting from a few weeks to a few years. The best way to handle it is to acknowledge it as a time of change and be gentle with yourself and your body and listen to and explore whatever new impulses begin to emerge, however kinky or odd they seem at the time. In my case celibacy was an awakening to spirituality, and it required I go into a state of seclusion so I could hear and give time to the new impulses awakening in me.

I believe celibacy is also necessary when one is breaking an addictive habit to sex or relationships, or as Nik Douglas says in Spiritual Sex, if one has difficulty believing that sex is a sacred act. What replaces addictive behaviour is the spiritual approach to life. What replaces a spiritual approach to life is addictive behaviour. Celibacy is like a cleansing fast – it can be just as nourishing at times in our lives to go without food for a time than to eat. When one takes the opportunity that celibacy offers to consolidate and examine one's erotic impulses and desires without the distraction and demands of a partner, one can emerge a clearer and more complete sexual being with renewed sexual energy.

Dolores French: I think it is very common for many couples to go through periods of not having sex and I feel it is one of the last sexual secrets. In most cases one of the people in the relationship has a problem and the other one doesn't. There are times when I don't feel like being sexual because of work, stress, illness, excitement and that is OK for me. There are times when I don't feel sexual, but these normally last a few hours as opposed to months at a time. When I am doing things with my family which involve my nieces and nephews I find that I become non-sexual, and can understand mothers feeling this way.

Candida Royalle: It can be very difficult when your lover is not interested in sex; it's difficult not to take it personally. Each one of us goes through times when we don't feel sexual. It does not mean that we do not love or desire our partner. If it goes on for a long time then there could be some problems which need to be addressed. It could be a time when you need to go into yourself and withdraw for a while. If you are a single person who does not want to have one-night stands, finding a good massage therapist is an essential ingredient because it is important to be touched and not lose that connection with our bodies and our sensuality. You need to find a way to be sensual with yourself.

Nina Hartley: I have had periods in my life with less sexual activity than others, but I have never been celibate, that is, voluntarily choosing to refrain from sexual activity with another person or myself. My job precludes me from being celibate, but when I'm away from my husband and wife (primarily when I'm on the road), I usually masturbate alone, even though opportunities for partner sex always present themselves.

If a person's decision to be celibate is a hysterical reaction to unresolved fears of sexuality, then it's merely a plaster applied to a severed artery. If it's deliberately used as a safe place from which to explore one's sexual issues, with intent to resolving them in order to live as a whole human being, then it's valuable. Celibacy in a relationship can only work with the agreement of all involved. One-sided celibacy in a relationship will only lead to loss of intimacy, anger, resentment and probable 'adulterous' behaviour in order to get basic needs met.

It's been my experience that celibate people are often on a spiritual trip, one that is alien to my sensibilities. I don't have anything against them, but I don't like to spend much time with them either. I find them concerned with subduing passion and desire and I'm all about the freeing of these energies.

Jo-Anne Baker: I think all relationships go through times when one or both people don't feel like having sex. I just think of it as a normal part of life. I believe we all have different needs. Our need to be loved can be expressed and received in many forms. If we focus on sex as the only way to experience closeness and intimacy we put a lot of pressure on ourselves and our partners. There have been long periods in my life when I was single and chose to use my sexual energy in creative ways in the world. There was a two-year period when I didn't make love to anyone; I spent time exploring Taoist and Tantric breath, and movement techniques and combined this with masturbation. I found it to be an invaluable time in being able to experience great depths of inner pleasure. By the time I met someone I wanted to be with our lovemaking became a new, exciting adventure which had a depth I had never experienced before.

Joani Blank: I respect people who are celibate, but it is not something that I am attracted to as I love being with people in a sexual way.

Ky: This is a time to make time for your own sexuality and find out what you like and what it does for you. I really like porn, so I would explore that. Don't put off satisfying yourself.

Minori Kitahara: I used to be afraid of being single and being in a relationship. When I was a single, I could not stand the loneliness. When I was in a relationship, I could not stand the restraints. Now, I understand whichever decision I make, I am what I am. The only difference between being single or in relationship is the amount of room you have in the bed. I am not interested in marriage. In Japan if women get married, they lose something important – freedom, pride, individuality. For many Japanese women, marriage means having no more dreams.

12

A Good Relationship

Everyone wants to know what makes a good relationship because we are not born with this knowledge, we learn it. Many people come from families that did not provide them with good relationship role models. It is not uncommon for children to grow up never seeing their parents expressing love to each other, or showing any displays of warmth, affection or touch. Often the reverse is commonplace and the home is a tense and hostile environment with emotionally absent parents. Often the idea of a good relationship comes from movies and television soap operas, which rarely mirror daily reality. The struggle of trying to balance financial stability and emotional security can cause much marital and relationship stress.

The 1960s shattered illusions about sexual roles, traditional marriage and what makes a good relationship. As women discovered their lack of personal and sexual satisfaction in their relationships they developed new ideas about what they wanted in their life. As women changed, so did the nature of their relationships.

Women who were in unhappy marriages left their domestic situations rather than 'putting up and shutting up' as their mothers might have done in the past. Women wanted a successful relationship at home, as well as in the workforce, with both places treating them with dignity, respect and reflecting her equality.

Our expectations of relationships have never been higher and are in some ways unrealistic. People now look for a soulmate, lover and friend in their partner and if the relationship is not an exciting place most of the time they vote with their feet and leave. Successful long-term relationships go through their ups and downs, and are distinguished by the commitment of both parties to work through issues.

A 'normal' relationship used to be a heterosexual marriage with a dominant male partner who was the breadwinner and a female partner who worked in the home and raised children. Today nothing could be further from the truth, with relationships encompassing every combination of personal sexual expression, ways of living, unusual domestic and financial relationships. This social diversity gives us the freedom to have more satisfying relationships.

While the women profiled in this book are known for their work in the area of sexuality, they have all had to deal with the same love and trust issues common to intimate relationships. For some of them their private lives have been enhanced by their public sex work and writings, while for others their private lives have had to carry the burden of their public notoriety. Their relationships and sexual identities cover every colour of the erotic rainbow, and their collective wisdom about what makes a good relationship is therefore invaluable.

Some of these women are polygamous, some are monogamous, and others have been celibate for years. Some of them have been in long-standing marriages, others in multiple marriages or open ones. Some are heterosexual, others bisexual, others lesbians. Some refuse to be bound by any sexual identity classification. But there are some things they all agree on: a good relationship is characterised by trust, honesty, friendship, and a willingness to let both parties change and grow. And, of course, love and sexual compatibility!

Annie Sprinkle: To have a good relationship you need to know yourself as well as possible, who you are and what you want. In my opinion, an ideal relationship is always based on being truthful, being able to be free to be yourself, and to be able to share your feelings. I think you should always tell your lover if you are having sex with someone else, even if it might end your relationship, because it is important to base your relationship on truth. (Unless your lover says she or he doesn't want to know.) Always share the truth in a loving way. Make a commitment never to be mean to your beloved, even if you are really, really angry. Do yell and scream all you want, but don't cross the line into being mean. Always stay loving to your lover, and your lover will stay loving to you.

Elizabeth Burton: Trust, similar interests, humour and communication.

Cora Emens: I am happy to be able to say that I have a good relationship with myself. I love myself and more and more I forgive myself. Actually, I quite like myself as a person: I am smart, playful, sexy, creative, friendly, short-tempered, stubborn and rebellious. I have learned to live with all my aspects instead of trying to get rid of certain parts of my character. Somehow it seems to work together, just as a rose isn't a real rose without the thorns on the stem.

You would not want to receive a rose from your lover without thorns, would you? So, since I love myself why shouldn't my partner love me?Sound egotistical to you? I am happy to say that my partner and I have a good relationship. We both independently came to the same conclusion: only if you love yourself can you accept that someone else can love you, too. Only if you can embrace yourself with all your flaws can you totally see through the rough bits of the 'other'.

Then love becomes easy. We can still enjoy a good fight every now and then, after all, a sense of truth has the right to be defended! But we've learned how to fight without really hurting each other. The fight becomes part of the game. A game, a challenge, perhaps, but not a threat. It is quite inspiring to get so passionately involved. We found great truths together this way. As long as you are willing to listen and respect your partner's viewpoint you cannot go wrong, you will love each other. As long as I or my partner can feel free to say whatever we think or desire, without the fear of being misunderstood, judged or insulted, we have a good relationship. It doesn't always mean that you can fulfil your partner's wishes or that your partner expects you to. Allowing each other the freedom to experience in life whatever is necessary for his or her personal growth is part of 'showing respect', 'having faith' and 'sharing'.

So my partner and I practise sharing with each other and our kids and in the meantime we improve the relationships we have with others. Some of them close, others more anonymous, like people we just meet. The relationships I have include myself, my lover, my daughters, my friends, the people I work with and all the people whom I have met and will meet in the future, nature, 'the spirit', my true self. What else? I am on my way... but it will take some more practice!

Jwala: Communication is the key to a good relationship. If you are holding back because of fear of expressing yourself it will affect how high and intense your ecstasy will be. The thing I have found to make my relationships work better is the ability to share and communicate and not withhold. I had a pattern of not saying anything when I was hurt or felt strange emotions, because I did not think I had the right to feel jealous. Now I express my feelings in words because it clears the air and I feel more intimate and present. Having clarification from the other person of what is going on with them brings us closer. To find an artform or technique to create harmony is the goal. If there is a misunderstanding or projection it needs to be cleared up as soon as possible.

Kutira: When you are truly happy within yourself, that's when you can really meet another person who would be right for you. If you come out of neediness, that you need somebody, then you're in trouble, because such a relationship is doomed to fail. When you love yourself totally, and are happy with yourself, totally, you can open yourself and love another. You come from a place of sustained fulfilment.

If I would have met Raphael, my husband, twenty years earlier in my life, we would not have made it. I had to first find that place of richness within. I wouldn't have had good communication skills, which is absolutely needed for any relationship that wants to thrive and grow. There may be a time to go through sexuality in an experimental way. But after a while your heart becomes more mature.

Loving yourself creates a mature heart that can create trust and rock-bottom commitments, the ability to make and sustain a commitment. And also, what I finally found was that I was running from intimacy. It was scary to commit to somebody my total being, all of who I am, the best and the worst; somebody who is not running away. Intimacy was the biggest step I had to take to allow myself to be vulnerable, and to show truly who I am. But in order to be fully intimate, you have to have the cornerstones of trust, integrity, commitment and truth. Like a pyramid, without the cornerstones it would fall down.

The other thing that seems to really work in our relationship is that we have boundaries. We are Tantra teachers, we are sensual with our friends and that opens up many doors. But Raphael and I are a committed monogamous couple and we totally honour that commitment. While I understand that each person and couple have their own choices to make about relationship boundaries, in our experience this works the best for us. We practise sex magic, and that's for Raphael and me and our love. That gives our Tantric relationship a sacred space to grow and blossom to its fullest.

Diane Torr: Don't judge your partner maliciously. Love with a full heart. Give of yourself eagerly. Be attentive to ways in which you can honour the love you share, such as spending an erotic weekend away from your day-to-day life. Give time and space in your life to explore your interest in each other. Strawberries dipped in chocolate used liberally.

norrie mAy-welby: Having been a partner to so many married people, and others whose main partners think they're monogamous, I've had to look at how realistic my personal fantasy of a monogamous relationship was. Of course, as a sex-positive activist, I maintain that monogamy is an option that is no more right or wrong than other options, generally speaking. And I've looked hard at whether my goals in intimate personal relationships are harmful, harmless, pleasure-producing, or someone else's ideas that I've absorbed as my own without them really serving me at all.

I've concluded that, for me, emotional commitment is much more important than physical monogamy, and I try to negotiate win-win rules where I can feel secure in a relationship while not restricting unnecessarily, or unrealistically, my partner's sexuality. Don't try to have someone else's relationship. Make your own. You are not your parents, nor are you someone in a movie or soap opera. Don't assume your partner has the same expectations you may bring to the relationship. Allow your relationship to be based on love and honesty, not on duty and covering up.

Be flexible and willing to negotiate and renegotiate the rules of your relationship, but make sure you respect your own bottom lines. Be willing to find what works for you, even if it may seem unusual or even 'wrong' by someone else's standards. This is your relationship, not your mother's.

Don't try to be everything for your partners, or insist that they depend only on you to meet their needs. It's only healthy for them to have friends and activities of their own, as it is for you. Allow each of you room to live and grow. A relationship should enhance your life, not replace it. Don't insist that this relationship be everything and forever. Be in the present with each other and yourself, not focused on tomorrow or yesterday.

Be gentle and play fair with each other. A relationship is not a competition to see whose will triumphs, or who is the most perfect wife/husband, girlfriend/boyfriend in the neighbourhood. Or at least, it shouldn't be seen as such a competition. The prize is not worth it.

Sometimes I have had to terminate relationships where my

bottom lines were not being met. This doesn't mean my partners were at fault, merely that they were not meeting my needs. It is not ultimately their responsibility to meet my needs – it is mine.

Never stay in a relationship out of fear, particularly fear of lack of love. Don't just give your partner love. Make sure you are giving yourself love too. The most important requirement of a good loving relationship with a partner is having a good loving relationship with yourself.

Shelly Mars: Communication. Constantly asking and talking about how you feel, and sharing this. It takes work and chemistry. Everybody has their secret demons inside, some people like to conquer and get somebody, and once they are conquered they have fear of abandonment. So they have to leave the relationship first, or they have to see someone else secretly. If you know yourself, and why you do these things, it helps.

Carol Queen: Mutual attraction, the ability to communicate, and the desire and willingness to make the relationship work are the basic necessities, I think. Love, too, of course, though sometimes romantic love is a problem, particularly when it leads to unrealistic expectations and an unwillingness to deal with change – romantic love is such a mainstay of many people's fantasies that it can be hard to focus on reality instead. Respect is as important as love and really, the two aren't entirely separate.

Ideally, I think a relationship should be able to balance the heady and overwhelming energy of romantic love plus lust (which has been termed 'l imerance') with something more stable – a focus on commitment to whatever the participants have decided is important. People who have chosen to be together need to be able to call upon the magic of their togetherness and still deal with the real world – disagree without bitterness, negotiate expectations, support each other's individuality as well as the relationship.

Note that I think any number of committed people can have this sort of relationship as a goal: two, of course, but also three or more. With each added partner the balance is more challenging to find and negotiation or communications skills are more critical, but I have seen long-term more-than-twosomes work.

Other factors include compatible senses of humour and mutual interests (at least, be very interested in each other as people, not only as lovers); compatible goals and standards around issues like work, money, offspring, monogamy and so forth. Sex, too, of course. A great relationship is one in which the participants like as well as love one another, are supportive as well as passionate.

Kimberly O'Sullivan: Love is not enough; you need a whole lot more going for you to keep two people together. Don't lie? ever. Always think of the consequences of any action on yourself, your partner and the relationship before you do it, not after the deed is done.

Relationships are a two-way street. Always ask 'Am I getting as much as I am giving?' Don't be a rescuer and don't be someone's mother. Make clear arrangements about relationship boundaries – what is emotionally okay with you, and what relationship behaviour crosses the boundaries of acceptability. Communicate this clearly.

If you really love someone don't walk out when the going gets tough. Most importantly, when you fall in love don't lose your friends, your own identity and your own life. Independence is essential to self-esteem.

Ruth Ostrow: Two people willing to compromise over and over and over again. Both with powerful senses of humour!

Rosie King: It is very important to accept and understand the gender differences in and out of the bedroom. Men and women are equal but definitely not the same – saying 'you're wrong and I'm right' is the sort of gender difference I am talking about. Men and women have different communication styles and differences in sexual needs and responses.

Sex needs to be put in context – it is not the be-all and end-all of life.

Sex in a relationship is like a glue and a lubricant; it is a glue because when sex is good it can bond the couple together and a lubricant because when things are tough a loving sex life can smooth over the rough edges of life.

I don't think that sex is the most important part of a relationship, however. When there are sexual difficulties it can poison even the best relationship. Sexual difficulties should be dealt with as soon as possible because they can be very toxic to the relationship. We all need to learn each other's language of love – everyone learns a specific language of love in the home they grow up in.

For some touch might be the way love is expressed and

experienced, or through words of love or gestures or spending time together. For example, when two people who speak different languages meet they are going to have to learn to speak each other's language or a common one. Otherwise they are not going to be able to communicate. It is exactly the same with the language of love – if your partner needs words of love then it is up to you to learn how to communicate love effectively.

For example, I need words of love, to be told that I am wonderful, lovely and beautiful, and I need plenty of touch and affection. My husband shows his affection by doing things for me and by spending time with me. This could be a recipe for disaster except that we both have learned to be bilingual and to value the other's language of love. It is very easy to say 'You don't love me', but it may be that your partner is expressing love in a way that you simply don't understand or value.

I don't think everyone has to have a relationship. That, again, is 'musterbation', but I do think that long-term relationships of all sorts are very important to us in increasing our self-awareness. If you want romance and chemistry in your long-term relationship you really have to work hard. Love in a relationship is like a rare tropical plant: if you don't feed and nurture it, it will die. Lord Wagner said, be a resident in your relationship, not a tourist. People think that they can be like absentee landlords, collecting rent from their relationships without maintaining the property. This is especially true of long-term romantic relationships. Because they are so intense, our partners are mirrors for us to look in to see who we are and these long-term relationships or marriages are crucibles. A crucible is a high-pressure, high-temperature vessel and if you put a metal into a crucible and heat it up it transforms the metal. I believe marriage does that. If you can stay the distance it can transform you into a much better person.

Tuppy Owens: Everyone has different needs but I would like to think that if people reversed their notion of a partner as someone they 'enjoy', 'own' or 'have' to someone they 'give pleasure to, including freedom to have sex with others' then the whole world would be a happier place. Relationships are best when they are wild and free. You don't have to dwell on when they might end, but bear in mind that permanence is unusual and so, not to be expected.

In Outsiders and my own life, it seems hard to strike the right balance between giving too much and not giving enough. But all you have to do is to discuss with your partner whether you're getting enough or not.

Amanda Dwyer: As far as relationships go, I have been married for many years to the same patient guy, whose constant support enables me to struggle through on days when I think I never want to speak to another male again. We had both been through previous relationships, which for various reasons resulted in divorce and a number of children. We made a commitment to each other that we both wanted our relationship to work. We continue to take that commitment seriously. I guess it is still the main reason why we remain together today.

During this time I have also been involved in a dominant-submissive relationship with a guy who is my dominant partner. I believe you need to be able to live both dominant and submissive roles to be good at either position. For some reason I don't understand, I continue to be involved with my dominant partner. I often believe it gives me a real-life balance while running Salon Kitty's. I do know it is connected to my work.

Without our personal commitment I doubt my husband would have persevered with my having this other relationship. Our commitment and trust keep holding us together. I believe they are the key elements to any successful relationship.

Cleo Dubois: There is no one simple answer to having a good relationship. What strikes me first as important is knowing yourself, knowing what you want, and being honest about it not only to your partner but to yourself. Ongoing communication is real work between partners. We now know that when we enter a relationship we bring to it not only our passion, our desire to love and to be loved, but also the luggage that our upbringings have burdened us with. In a sense, both partners bring to the relationship their own parents and the cultural norms and expectations they grew up with.

We need to sort out our issues so that we can know and understand what our needs are and have a chance to find fulfilment in some way. For me, a good relationship must be deeply rooted in heart space and love. As for sexual compatibility, two people can rarely fulfil all of each other's needs. We look for working compromises and agreements. It is possible to be an ethical 'slut' and there are many ways to negotiate this, such as consensual, selective non-monogamy. Parity and priorities are really important to pay attention to and this can be a delicate balancing act for both partners.

Exploring the boundaries of our sexuality, perhaps even across gender lines, having friends with whom we share some aspects of our sexuality, certainly enriches us and allows us to live our sexual lives to the full, at least some of the time.

Kat Sunlove: Communicate and forgive.

Deborah Sundahl: Know thyself. Communicate thyself. Listen to what is being said and acknowledge it without attachment to what it may or may not mean to you.

Dolores French: Statistics show that medically and emotionally marriage is good for men, but divorce is good for women. Right before one of my marriages, I gave my attorney a small retainer on handling a future divorce settlement. He said, 'This doesn't seem very optimistic'. I said, 'Get real. Marriage is the first step to divorce'. A few years later my husband tried to retain him for a divorce. I'm glad I had planned ahead. I've had the same attorney through five marriages now. My most recent marriage has lasted eleven years and looks good for lasting quite a few more. Does practice really make perfect?A friend of mine was furious when he came home unannounced from a business trip and found his girlfriend in bed with another guy. I told my friend that, 'If you want people to live up to your expectations, you usually have to provide them with the script, the props and the cues'. He had never specifically told her that he didn't want to find her in bed with another guy and no arrangement had been made to avoid the offending scene. Instead of renegotiating, he chose to end their relationship.

Relationships are not sting operations. Often people believe that if they can manipulate their partners into an agreement, it's a done deal, no matter how unlikely it is that such an agreement can be kept.

Candida Royalle: Communication and respect for your partner as well as taking responsibility for your own actions. Being compassionate to one another but before you get to that place I think it really helps to have a strong sense of who you are.

Nan Kinney: I have no clue. My girlfriend will attest to this. But seriously, it's communication. The same as with sex, it all comes down to communication. (Taking out the garbage doesn't hurt either.) You cannot be afraid to express yourself. You have to be able to speak and to listen. You have to want to know how the other person's doing, to be attuned to each other's feelings. And you have to be assertive about those feelings too; you cannot just hear something is wrong and then not be willing to address it or do something about it.

For example, I'm in a relationship now where my girlfriend was in a job that she hated and she needed to talk about it every night. So I not only needed to listen to her feelings of unhappiness and fear and low self-esteem, but also try to come up with a way to work it out. To try to help her out of it. Relationships are not static; they're always changing and you have to be okay with that. She finally left her job, but that was after many nights of sitting up late and her waking up in the middle of the night crying because she knew she had to leave the place that was making her crazy.

Respect is key. You have to respect the other person's individuality. Guard your lover's solitude, as Rilke wrote. So many lesbians just seem to become one, which often results in lesbian bed death. You need to keep your own interests, your own friends, your solitude or alone time, so you can continue to bring something to the relationship.

For example, I work out and run every morning for about an hour. That's where I can be alone and have my own thoughts. We try to make time for each other to have the apartment to herself. We have mutual friends and separate friends. It's not a big deal if one of us goes out and the other one stays home and watches TV.

Your lover is a real live person, not just another part of you. That takes work. I've had to work at it very hard. You have to be secure in yourself, and do things that help you to feel secure. You have to like yourself, which is a problem for many women. You have to do things that make you feel good about yourself. That's why I run every day. I begin each day feeling good about myself.

Nina Hartley: I know from personal experience it's not possible to have a truly good relationship without self-esteem and self-love. I've learned that one inflicts pain on others because one is feeling pain. If necessary, get therapy to resolve that primal pain and injury. If you do not love yourself, you can not permit anyone of quality to love you, and you will sabotage all relationships.

Without self-respect, you will treat others badly, or will permit them to mistreat you while thinking you deserve it. Without self-esteem, you can only be servile toward others who show you kindness, not let their kindness or love heal you; you will be subservient to get their attention but will not be able to be submissive to your heart.

Jo-Anne Baker: There are three main ingredients for having a good relationship.

Be affectionate with one another every day – cuddle before you go to sleep or when you wake up. Hold hands and touch one another in a non-sexual way. Often couples form a pattern when the only time they touch is when one of them wants sex. Problems arise when one of them does not want to have sex. Creating more intimacy in relationships starts with physical contact that is sensual and caring.

Say nice things to one another every day, expressing your appreciation and love for your partner is an essential ingredient.

Initially it feels strange to say, 'I really appreciate the care you took in doing... for me', 'I love you', 'You look sexy tonight', 'I think you are wonderful/gorgeous/beautiful/ handsome'.

After you start to compliment your partner you can see how he or she is able to relax and feel happy. It also encourages your partner to compliment you. For very busy people leaving 'love' messages on the answering machine or notes is a creative way to remain connected.

Spend quality time together every week doing something that you both enjoy. Many couples start to drift apart after a while because they have nothing in common. Taking up a new hobby or activity is a way of expanding your interests together. Spending time together in nature is a wonderful way to relax and unwind as is getting dressed up and going somewhere special together.

Most of us fantasise about the ideal partner, but if we manifested a replica of what we wanted, or ourselves, within a short period of time we would be arguing and discontented.

I also believe relationships are there for us to grow and are often a challenge because they cause us to look at ourselves, which can be painful. Remembering that we are doing the best we can is a way of being compassionate with one another, when we are going through difficult times. Learning and putting into practice how to love another on a deep level is something that goes on until the day we die.

Joani Blank: Many people get into talking about their relationship as a way to avoid talking about sex. You can pay lots of attention to your relationship, but the real problem is a sexual one. Sex is always interactive. Anyone you are having sex with you are having a relationship with, even if it is only a one-night stand.

One book I would like to write is 'No More Secret Affairs', with the emphasis on the 'secret', not the 'affair'. It would not be a book about how not to have affairs, but a book on how to manage non-monogamy. The particular form of non-monogamy that is commonly practised in the US is where the couple are in a committed relationship but one or both partners are having sex with someone else either occasionally or on an ongoing basis. Statistics show that this occurs in two-thirds of relationships.

Typically what happens is that the man is caught out and he swears he will never do it again – which he may or may not – and they go on to live miserably ever after. Or at least he does, because he likes to have affairs. The alternative is that the relationship ends. They are the only two options most people have. There is not the alternative 'Let's see how we can work this out in a way so that we can have sex with other people and it doesn't damage our relationship'. I would like to interview couples who can successfully negotiate this for a reasonable length of time.

Ky: Communication and humour are the two most important things. Your partner should be your love star. I run a business with my partner of six years, and it could have finished us because we are so different, but we have instead negotiated a great personal-work split. In a relationship you have to acknowledge normal feelings like fear and insecurity.

Minori Kitahara: Don't think you have to be nice to everybody. Love yourself.

Contacts

Jo-Anne Baker: For mail order sexual products and individual sessions contact The Pleasure Spot, PO Box 213, Woollahra NSW 2025, tel: (02) 9361 0433, fax: (02) 9331 6120, email: pleasurepot@ozemail.net

Joani Blank: Website at http://www.joaniblank.com

Tracy Cox: Website at http://www.tracycox.com. Tracy can be contacted c/o Anglia TV, Norwich, NR1 3JG

Cléo Du Bois: Website: http://www.cleodubois.com

Cora Emens: New Ancient Sex Academy, alex. Boersstraat 30 sous, 1071 KZ, Amsterdam, tel: (0) 20 6644670

Websites at http://www.willemderidder.com and http://come.to/coracoracora, email: cora@flash.A2000.nl.

Nina Hartley: Website: http://www.nina.com

Jwala: For Jwala's workshops contact Good Vibrations, San Francisco, USA, tel: (415) 974 8990, fax: (415) 974 8989, email: goodvibe@well.com.

Nan Kinney: Fatale videos available through Good Vibrations, San Francisco, US, tel: (415) 974 8990, fax: (415) 974 8989, website: http://www.goodvibes.com

Minori Kitahara: Love Piece Club, Japan, tel: (813) 5226 9072, fax: (813) 5226 9093, email: love@ummit.co.jp, website: http://www.ummit.co.jp/~lovc.

Kutira: To receive newsletters and teaching schedules, or to order audio tapes or CD's contact Kahua Hawaiian Institute, PO Box 1747, Makawao, HI 96768, USA, tel: (808) 572 6006, fax: (808) 572 0088, email: kahua@OceanicTantra.com, web: http://www.OceanicTantra.com.

Ky: Sh!, 39 Coronet Street, London, NI 6HD, UK, tel: (0207) 613

5458, fax: (0207) 613 0020, web: www.sh!-womenstore.co.uk.

norrie mAy-Welby: Website at http://www.cat.org.au/ultra/ultra1.html.

Linda Montano: For information about lectures, performance workshops, residencies, tours and Art/Life Counselling, write to The Art/Life Institute, 185 Abeel Street, Kingston, NY 12401, USA.

Tuppy Owens: For information about Outsiders, Sex Maniac's Ball and the Sexual Freedom Coalition, contact Tuppy at PO Box 4ZB, London W1A 44ZB, UK, fax: (0207) 493 4479. Donations welcome. *Planet Sex - The Handbook* costs US$25 (cheques to T. Owens).

Carol Queen: Carol's videos and books can be bought through Good Vibrations, San Francisco, US, tel: (415) 974 8990, fax: (415) 974 8989, website: http://www.goodvibes.com

Candida Royalle: Website at http://www.royalle.com.

Deborah Sundal: Deborah's videos on female ejaculation are available through Good Vibrations, San Francisco, US, tel:(415) 974 8990, fax: (415) 974 8989, website: http://www.goodvibes.com

Annie Sprinkle: Annie's products can be ordered through Gates of Heck US, tel: (212) 879 5016 and Good Vibrations, San Francisco, US, tel: (415) 974 8990, fax: (415) 974 8989,
website: http://www.goodvibes.com

Veronica Vera: Miss Vera's Finishing School For Boys Who Want To Be Girls, PO Box 1331, Old Chelsea Station, New York, NY 10011, USA, tel: (212) 242 6449, fax (212) 242 2273, email: webhostess@missvera.com, web: www.missvera.com. To receive a copy of Veronica Vera's book, write to 85 Eighth Avenue, New York, NY 10011, USA.

Books, videos and multimedia

Women Sex Performance Artists

John Heidenry, *What Wild Ecstasy: The Rise and Fall of the Sexual Revolution*, Simon & Schuster, 1997.

Lucinda Jarrett, *Stripping in Time: A History of Erotic Dancing*, Pandora/HarperCollins, 1997.

Annie Sprinkle, *Herstory Of Porn - Reel to Real*, video, 1998 (available through The Pleasure Spot, tel: (02) 9361 0433, fax: (02) 9331 6120).

Post-Porn Modernist: My 25 Years as a Multimedia Whore, Cleis Press, 1998.

The Sluts and Goddess Video Workshop: Or How to Be a Sex Goddess in 101 Easy Steps, video, 1992 (available through The Pleasure Spot, tel: (02) 9361 0433, fax: (02) 9331 6120).

Spiritual Sexuality

Margo Anand, *The Art of Sexual Magic: How to Use Sexual Energy to Transform Your Life*, Piatkus, London, 1995.

Ancient Secrets of Sexual Ecstasy for Modern Lovers, video, 1996 (available through Good Vibrations, tel: (415) 974 8990, fax: (415) 974 8989, email: goodvibe@well.com).

Cynthia Connop (director), *Sacred Sex*, video, Tantric Arts Pty Ltd, 1995 (available through The Pleasure Spot, tel: (02) 9361 0433, fax: (02) 9331 6120).

Nik Douglas, *Spiritual Sex: Secrets of Tantra From the Ice Age to the New Millennium*, Pocket Books, New York, 1997.

Jwala, *Sacred Sex: Ecstatic Techniques for Empowering Relationships*, Mandala, California, 1993.

Gender Bending

Kate Bornstein, *My Gender Workbook*, Routledge, New York & London, 1998.

Pat Califia, *Sex Changes: The Politics of Transgenderism*, Cleis Press, 1997.

Carolyn Dinshaw & David M. Halperian (eds), GLQ: *A Journal of Lesbian and Gay Studies*, vol. 4, no. 4, 1998.

Leslie Feinberg, *Stone Butch Blues*, Firebrand Books, New York, 1993.

Veronica Vera, *Miss Vera's Finishing School For Boys Who Want To Be Girls: Tips, Tales, and Teaching from the Dean of the World's First Cross-Dressing Academy*, Doubleday, New York, 1997.

Women Scribes and Educators

Jill Julius Matthews (ed.), *Sex in Public: Australian Sexual Cultures*, Allen & Unwin, Sydney, 1997.

Susan Mitchell, *Icons, Saints and Divas*, HarperCollins, Sydney, 1997.

Kimberly O'Sullivan, *Magazines Kink*, Wicked Women Publications, Sydney, 1991.

Ruth Ostrow, *Burning Urges*, Pan Macmillan, Sydney, 1997.

Hot and Sweaty, Pan Macmillan, Sydney, 1997.

Carol Queen, *Exhibitionism For The Shy*, Down There Press, San Francisco, 1995.

Real Live Nude Girl: Chronicles of Sex-Positive Culture, Cleis Press, 1997.

Sallie Tisdale, *Talk Dirty to Me: An Intimate Philosophy of Sex*, Pan Books, London, 1994.

Richard Wherrett (ed.), *Mardi Gras!: True Stories from Lock Up to Frock Up*, Viking Books, Sydney, 1999.

Physical Challenges

Rosie King, *Good Loving Great Sex: Finding Balance When Your Sex Drives Differ*, Random House, Sydney, 1997.

Ken Kroll & Erica Levy Klein, *Enabling Romance: A Guide to Love, Sex and Relationships for Disabled*, Crown Publishers/Harmony Books, 1992.

Joan Nestle, *A Fragile Union*, Cleis Press, 1999.

Tuppy Owens, *The Outsiders Club: Practical Suggestions*, self-published, London, 1990.

Sex After 50, video, 1991 (available through Good Vibrations, tel: (415) 974 8990, fax: (415) 974 8989, email: goodvibe @well.com).

Domination and Submission

Gloria Brame, *Different Loving: An Exploration of the World of Sexual Domination and Submission*, Random House/Villard Books, 1993.

Pat Califia & Drew Campbell (eds), *Bitch Goddess: The Spiritual Path of the Dominate Woman*, Greenery Press, 1997.

Cléo Dubois, *Fetish*, CD-ROM, Edge Interactive, 1996.
Jay Wiseman, *S & M* 101, Greenery Press, 1996.

Female Ejaculation and Oral Sex

Jacqueline and Steve Franklin, *The Ultimate Kiss*, Media Products, 1982.

Dolores French, *Working*, E.P. Dutton, New York, 1988.

Debra Sundhal, videos on female ejaculation (available through Good Vibrations, tel: (415) 974 8990, fax: (415) 974 8989, email: goodvibe@well.com).

Cathy Winks, *Good Vibrations Guide: The G-Spot*, Down There Press, San Francisco, 1998.

Film and Pornography

Nina Hartley, *Deep Inside*, video, 1993 (available through Good Vibrations, tel: (415) 974 8990, fax: (415) 974 8989, email: goodvibe@well.com).

Robert Rimmer (ed.), *X-Rated Videotape Guides*, vols 1, 2 and 3, Prometheus Books, 1986, 1991, 1993.

Robert J. Stoller, *Porn: Myths for the Twentieth Century*, Yale University Press, 1991.

Robert J. Stoller & I. S. Levine, *Coming Attractions: The Making of an X-Rated Video*, Yale University Press, 1993.

Women's Sex Shops

Joani Blank (ed.), *First Person Sexual: Women and Men Write About Self-pleasuring*, Down There Press, San Francisco, 1996.

Good Vibrations: The Complete Guide To Vibrators, Down There Press, San Francisco, 1989.

Cathy Winks & Anne Semans, *The New Good Vibrations Guide To Sex*, Cleis Press, 1997.

Jay Wiseman, *Sex Toy Tricks: More than 125 Ways to Accessorize Good Sex*, Greenery Press, 1996.

Women With Women

Susie Bright, *Sexwise*, Cleis Press, 1995.